Newborn Mothers

WHEN A BABY IS BORN,
SO IS A MOTHER.

by *Julia Jones*

Newborn Mothers – When a Baby is Born, so is a Mother.

ISBN: 978-0-6483431-2-7 (hardcover)
ISBN: 978-0-6483431-4-1 (paperback)
ISBN: 978-0-6483431-3-4 (eBook)

Book cover design: Michelle Mildenberg
Book layout: eMatti
Printed on demand and distributed by IngramSpark

Keywords:
        Newborn Mothers
        Babies
        Julia Jones

Contents

Acknowledgment of Country

I acknowledge the traditional custodians of the land where I write this book, the Whadjak Nyungar people, and pay my respects to their elders past, present and future. I would like to extend this acknowledgement to the first nations people of the world, wherever you may be reading this book.

Dedication

This book is for you, Newborn Mother. Written in appreciation of your efforts to raise happy, healthy children and create a better future. In recognition of all the invisible work you do, both internally and out in the world, every day and every night.

I thank you for taking time out of your full life to read this book. I promise to do my best to make good use of your time and I hope that this book will ultimately give you more time, more freedom, more peace and more joy. I want you to enjoy every page of this book and walk away feeling inspired.

Your Free Audiobook

Together we can change the world! To thank you for buying this book and being part of the renaissance my gift to you is a free audiobook.

I know how precious your time is so I've read and recorded this entire book for you to listen to you whilst you keep your eyes on your toddler, take a walk in the sunshine or relax in the bath. Multi-tasking is what mums do best!

This free gift is available for download for people who purchase this ebook or printed book only by entering your email at

www.newbornmothers.com/audiobook.

Introduction

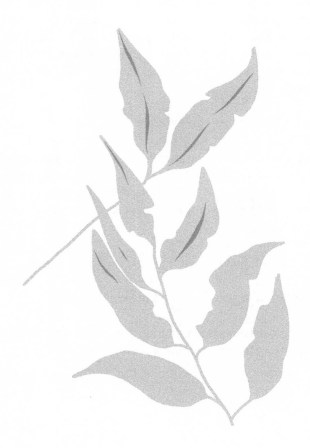

About This Book

The challenges we face as women on our journey to motherhood are complex and require solutions at many levels. There are external barriers to our motherhood happiness, like discrimination at work, gender bias in medicine and research, expensive and poor-quality childcare and lack of paid parental leave. These changes need to happen at a more global level.

That's not what this book is about.

Newborn Mothers is for mothers who want to take action on an individual level in their own lives. As you expand your life in peace and joy, you are inviting other mothers to join you in peace and joy too. Together, we can create a new blueprint for motherhood.

This is a manifesto for an internal revolution.

A revolution in your heart and in your home.

This book is your invitation to join the renaissance of a more joyful, peaceful transformation to motherhood.

A Note on Postpartum

You say postnatal, I say postpartum. What's the difference anyway?

Post simply means 'after', *partum* and *natal* both mean 'birth'.

While they are synonyms for the period just after a baby is born, there is a subtle difference. *Partum* refers to the one giving birth (i.e. the mother) and *natal* refers to the one being birthed (i.e. the baby).

Postnatal is the term more commonly used here in Australia, whereas *postpartum* is used more in the United States. This is one of the few times I jump the fence with my language. I choose to use *postpartum* as it more accurately reflects my mission to support mothers, and to remedy the gap I see in our culture of care.

However, if you are more familiar with the term postnatal, it could be used interchangeably with the word postpartum throughout this book, without altering the meaning.

A Note on Gender

Unfortunately, the English language lacks gender-neutral pronouns. I love the word mother as a powerful feminine archetype and therefore refer to the birthing parent as she. For clarity, I then refer to the baby as he.

I acknowledge that some readers may not identify with these genders and hope you can still find value in this book.

They Smile Just in Time

Just when you are on the verge of listing your baby on eBay — "free to a good home" — a miraculous thing happens.

He smiles.

Oh, joy of joys!! The only thing more loveable than a sleeping baby is a smiling baby.

But here's the catch: for your baby to learn to smile, you need to learn to smile too.

The Numbers

One in seven women in Australia will experience postnatal depression. That's 48,400 women — enough to fill 116 jumbo jets — every year.[1]

More than two-thirds of mothers do not meet their own breastfeeding goals. These are not goals set by the government or the World Health Organization. These are goals set by the kind and generous mothers themselves, who want to feed their baby, and don't have the support they need.[2]

Marriages suffer during the transition to parenthood. As early as 1957, psychologist Edward LeMasters published a paper claiming that becoming parents caused a marriage crisis. Back then, he was ridiculed. This was supposed to be the happiest time of your life! But decades of research since have shown consistently that conflict increases dramatically in marriages once a baby is introduced.[3]

And the leading cause of maternal death in Australia is suicide.[1]

This is not a problem unique to one part of the world. You can research the numbers in almost any industrialised nation and they will paint a similar picture.

Women are suffering. Babies are suffering. Marriages are suffering. Something has gone terribly wrong, if this suffering is how we are experiencing what should be the most joyful time of our lives.

The Start of Something

I didn't know all those numbers when I started out as a postpartum doula at only 24 years old, before I was even a mother myself. I came to postpartum work through my interest in Ayurveda, traditional Indian medicine. When I learned about Ayurvedic postpartum care, I knew this was my calling in life.

Over the next few years I studied five different postpartum doula trainings, and while they were all excellent in their own ways, none of them really got much deeper than practical information about baby care and breastfeeding.

None of them really addressed how to support Newborn Mothers through this major life transition, this rite of passage.

None of them acknowledged the deep and profound changes going on inside a Newborn Mother's brain, let alone how we — as professionals — could support them through it.

5

Although I started my doula business, providing massage and meals for Newborn Mothers, I knew there was something more. When I had my own first baby, the need to find answers became even more urgent.

I started exploring postpartum from different perspectives including through my own background in social justice and community development. I dove into newer areas of study to me, from anthropology to evolution, traditional medicine to brain science, and eventually pulled together a radically new paradigm for postpartum transformation.

Now, over a decade later, my work has evolved. I've written books and created online courses, available worldwide, for Newborn Mothers and the professionals who work with them.

The Faces

When I first began working as a postpartum doula, I received many emails. Even though I worked, at that time, only in my local area, these emails came from exhausted and overwhelmed mothers all over the world.

These are the faces behind the numbers: the individual Newborn Mothers who are suffering; the stories that the statistics don't quite show.

"I have three children under four years old, and have certainly gone through my share of desperation, depression, and feelings of total failure. Motherhood has rocked my world." — Bri

"I am almost in tears. I am a mother of a one-and-a-half-year-old and three-and-a-half-year-old. My transition into

parenthood for my first baby was extremely difficult. Birth was healthy, baby was healthy, breastfeeding was normal... but it was still the hardest transition in my entire life."
— Samantha

"I have felt so saddened that with both of my babies the circumstances of my life and conditioning of my culture prevented me from fully experiencing that sacred window of time in the way that I wanted. I feel so exhausted and stretched thin caring for my five-month-old and my two-year-old. I have found myself feeling resentful when my little ones won't nap, or my husband wants to be close." — Nara

Hearing so many women's stories, I began to see patterns. Many mothers found ways to excuse their suffering, almost apologising that they were not enjoying motherhood, as though the problem was unique to them.

It was hard for me because of colic.

Things would have been different if I hadn't had a traumatic birth.

If only my family lived closer...

I shouldn't have had my babies so close in age.

There are a million reasons why it might be intense for you — often more intense than giving birth — but none of them is entirely true. The truth is it's intense for nearly all of us.

And surely this points to some broader cultural systemic problem making mothers feel desperate and depleted.

7

It's not your individual circumstances.

And it's not any shortcomings as a mother.

And it's certainly not your fault.

"But These are the Best Days of Your Life"

Any time you complain about any aspect of mothering, you are likely to be told to enjoy it, because "they grow up so fast".

Retrospectively, it seems like a blink of the eye. But while the years may fly by, the days are long and the nights are longer.

Maybe living in the moment works for some mothers, but often when you express your struggle, what you're really looking for is acknowledgment of your emotions, your experience.

In that moment, it doesn't feel like it *will* pass. At 3am, there is no light at the end of the tunnel. Maybe you feel like the darkness goes on forever.

"But these are the best days of your life" is society's narrowly defined script for mothers, and it prevents us from agitating, from making change.

Instead, it feels more like *A Tale of Two Cities*: "It was the best of times, it was the worst of times."

As a parent, the highs are higher than you ever experienced before you had children. But the lows are also lower. The happiness scale got rearranged. There are more extremes of emotion; nothing is steady or familiar.

There is more boredom, loneliness, suffering. But there is also more joy, peace and bliss.

Your baby enjoying his first heart-melting giggle. Watching your partner soothe your baby to sleep. Savouring that rare hot cup of tea, alone.

Those transcendent moments are what keep you going, refuel you until the next pit stop, whenever the hell that will be.

How long is Postpartum?

Postpartum is generally recognised as the six weeks after birth. Medicine, science, and traditional cultures around the world acknowledge that this is a unique time in a woman's life requiring specific care.

But since postpartum literally means *after birth*, you could consider a woman postpartum for the rest of her life! I believe we need to expand our understanding of postpartum and prefer to see it in stages, unfolding in layers over time and requiring longer term emotional and practical support.

Mothers commonly ask me how long postpartum lasts, usually because they are convinced they should have 'bounced back' by now. I'll let you in on something right from the start... there is no 'back to normal' after you have a baby, because becoming a mother alters the very structure of your brain and you will never be the same person you once were.

9

This can be a great opportunity indeed! You are being invited to reinvent yourself, because when a baby is born, so is a mother.

And let me tell you the truth... *the birth of a mother can be more intense than childbirth.*

Postpartum ≠ Depression

Contrary to pop culture use, postpartum does not mean depression. Postpartum is the time after birth, and postpartum depression is when depression is experienced during this time.

Sadly, depression is the experience of so many women at this stage of their lives that the word *postpartum* has become synonymous with depression. And perhaps with the stigma around mental health, some people feel more comfortable avoiding the use of words like *depression* and *anxiety*, and find it easier to say, "I had postpartum" or "I've got postnatal".

I'd like to see the word *postpartum* reclaimed to reflect it's true meaning — an opportunity for profound personal transformation.

This transformation can be positive or negative, largely depending on the way your community supports or neglects Newborn Mothers.

And once we have an understanding of the impact that this time can have on women and babies and families and the whole community, it becomes critical that we give mothers the support they need during what my teacher Ysha Oakes called "a Sacred Window of Time".

"After birth, there is a Sacred Window of time; a time for complete rejuvenation of a woman's physical, mental and spiritual health. A time for deep, extended bonding with her newborn. The first 42 days after birth set the stage for her next 42 years." — Ysha Oakes

What is a Newborn Mother?

The process of becoming a mother is gradual, not abrupt, and I use the term Newborn Mother to reflect this state of profound transformation, no matter how long ago your baby was born, or how many babies you have.

You can feel like a Newborn Mother whether or not your baby is biologically related to you, and whether or not you are actively mothering your child.

If you can relate to this transformation — this idea of being born as a mother — then you are a Newborn Mother.

Being a Newborn Mother lasts as long as you need to become confident and strong.

Newborn Mother —

A recently born mother, whose strength is asking for help. She acknowledges that the birth of a mother is more intense than childbirth, and that she is as sensitive and vulnerable as her baby. Her heart is wide open and her needs are high. As she nourishes herself, she nourishes her children.

If you are a Newborn Mother, then this book is for you.

11

Transformation

Transformation is a buzz word these days, but truly there is no greater transformation than motherhood. Painful and powerful, it stretches you to your limits… and beyond.

Transformation involves rebirth, which also involves loss. There are deep internal shifts in ways of knowing and understanding the world around you. Maybe you are grieving as your old self is gone, superseded. Maybe you feel as though you almost don't exist.

Motherhood truly changes you, from the inside out. I mean this quite literally. Often, when a pregnant woman thinks about having a baby, she thinks of herself *plus* a new baby.

Rarely do we realise that there will be a new self too. A newborn baby. And a Newborn Mother.

Artist Sarah Walker described becoming a mother as "like discovering the existence of a strange new room in the house where you already live".[4]

It sounds poetic, and it's true, even on a very basic biological level.

Among many other changes, the structure and even size of your brain alters when you have a baby…

Your Brain

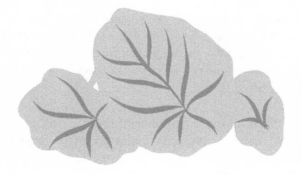

Introducing Your New Brain

For too long, science was the domain of men. Yet when we have a woman's perspective, it can dramatically alter our understanding of a subject.

Marian Diamond was one such pioneer.[1]

Born in 1926, Marian was an anatomical neuroscientist who studied the impact of environmental factors on brain development. Until then, it was thought that the human brain was largely fixed by genetics and unchangeable. Her research compared the brains of rats that experienced 'enriched' (stimulated) or 'impoverished'(unstimulated) environmental conditions in their cages. Her major scientific contributions to neuroplasticity — the brain's ability to adapt to change by forming new pathways — have changed how we view the human brain.

In the 1970s, Marian, a mother of four, wanted to research how the female brain changed during the transition to motherhood. Rats are commonly used for research because their brains function in a surprisingly similar way to humans. At the time, there was a strong bias towards using only male rats in research to avoid the way that female hormonal fluctuations might affect the data. (Actually, we know now that female rats vary no more than male rats do.[4; 5; 6; 7])

Unusually for her time, Marian put a range of rats — male, female, pregnant and non-pregnant — through enrichment programs with wheels, mazes, tunnels and toys. The rats in these enriched environments consistently demonstrated growth in their cerebral cortex, which in turn caused better performance in navigating mazes. Another group of rats were kept in bare cages, and their brains did not change in these impoverished environments.

However, there was one exception. The brains of the rats who were pregnant during their time spent in enriched or impoverished cages did not exhibit the same change as the brains of the male or non-pregnant female rats. The pregnant rats, who were mothers by this stage, had the same sized cortex whether or not they'd been in impoverished or enriched environments.

Imagine Marian's shock!

Does this mean pregnant women and new mothers cannot learn? That our brains cannot change and improve? Maybe they were right all along and mothers are good for nothing but domesticity.

But on closer examination, Marian realised that the pregnancy itself had been an enrichment for the female rat brain, stimulating it and leading to a thicker cerebral cortex.[3] She postulated that pregnancy stimulated the brain and that therefore motherhood is an enrichment program. Their brains didn't change, because they were already changed.

Marian made this discovery way back in 1971, but it was largely ignored. The notion of neuroplasticity has only very recently become recognised in popular culture.

The development of more sophisticated research techniques like functional magnetic resonance imaging has allowed scientists to take a much closer look at these changes in living human brains. One study in 2017 showed a significant reduction in brain volume following pregnancy that lasted

15

for around two years. In fact, the changes that happen in our brains during pregnancy are so consistent that a computer algorithm can tell with 100% accuracy if a woman has been pregnant just from an MRI scan.[2]

These results suggest an adaptive process for women in the transition to motherhood, which, interestingly, was shown to occur regardless of whether the means of conception was natural or due to fertility treatment.[2] The study also speculated that it is these pregnancy-related brain changes that may contribute to the memory reduction often experienced in pregnancy[2] and also known as 'baby brain'.

Baby Brain

Women in the mothers groups I run frequently ask if other new mothers also feel really stupid since having their babies. One mother in particular said that she is so forgetful, emotional, sensitive and unable to concentrate that her husband even told her she used to be smarter than she is now!

'Baby brain', 'mummy brain' or 'pregnancy brain' are generally considered insults in our masculine culture. There is a long history of women being deemed hysterical, crazy and even mentally ill for being empathetic and compassionate, or unhappy with the status quo. Is baby brain an elaborate story we tell women to keep them in the kitchen? Or is there a biological basis?

Exploring the brain, and especially women's brains, is a growing field. There is very little known about the effects of pregnancy on the human brain.[5] Pregnancy-related cognitive and memory decline tends to be overstated in popular culture and the term 'baby brain' is usually used in a derogatory way, but when we take a closer look there are fascinating and hugely *positive* side effects of becoming a mother. It's time we understood and celebrated the unique brilliance of our feminine brains.

"There is growing evidence that pregnancy and lactation are associated with a variety of alterations in neural plasticity, including adult neurogenesis, functional and structural synaptic plasticity, and dendritic remodeling in different brain regions. All of the mentioned changes are not only believed to be a prerequisite for the proper fetal and neonatal development, but moreover to be crucial for the physiological and mental health of the mother."[4]

I use the term 'baby brain' as an act of subversion, to represent the ways our brains change to prepare us and protect us during the transition to motherhood. I'm going to show you how embracing baby brain is one of the secrets to finding the peace and joy you are longing for in motherhood.

"When Julia explained baby brain to me, it empowered me to consider all that I have managed to achieve over the last seven weeks! The pressure of realising I haven't become dumb or inadequate has been released and I feel invigorated that my brain is doing what it needs to do to care for me and my baby." — Jessica

"Learning about the baby brain haze we're designed to bliss out in has been so freeing. It feels deliciously wise and counter-cultural to focus purely on restoration and nurturing. I'm learning to work with my body and not against it and I notice I'm growing too." — Alexa

17

"The stigma attached to baby brain (and early motherhood overall) has robbed many women of such a profound experience. It's absolutely time to change that and see the positive shift that happens in society as a result." — Katilin

There are a number of changes that occur in your brain when you are born as a mother. I'm going to focus on two of them. The first is increased neuroplasticity, meaning your brain is able to change and is open to *learning*. The second is increased production and receptivity to oxytocin, which rewires your brain for more *loving*. It's a combination of these factors (and, let's face it, sleep deprivation) that I call baby brain.

Let's take a look.

Learning

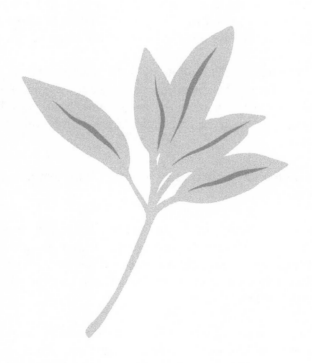

Plasticity

In our culture, we tend to romanticise motherhood to the point of fetishism. As though when we give birth, women instantly know exactly how to care for their new babies and find complete life satisfaction in that role alone. We think of mothering as an innate ability, specific to women.

But mothering — and fathering and care-giving in general — is a learned skill. And learning new skills requires time, patience and practice. It's totally okay if you don't know what to do straight away. Fortunately, nature prepared your brain beautifully for this period of intense learning.

As I touched on, neuroplasticity is the adaptive ability of the brain to form and reorganise in response to its environment. When you have a baby, it makes sense that your brain plasticity increases in preparation for learning how to be a mother.[3]

But we face a problem when we try to learn feminine skills in a masculine way.

Ideally, we would not be limited by our gender or sex. I believe we each have the capacity to tune in to the masculine and feminine *archetypes* within ourselves, each of which I will elaborate on in the next section, and each of which is useful at different stages.

Becoming a parent is a good time to tune in to the mother archetype within you. In general, though, our culture favours a more masculine approach to tackling most of life's problems and opportunities.

Information Frenzy

As a child, you were probably prepared for life in a masculine world. I hope you were raised to believe that girls could do anything that boys can do, like going to school and having a career. In your old life, you were measured against masculine indicators of success, like being competitive and independent and logical.

Information was power and everything was figure-outable — just ask guru Google!

But what happens when you've spent your whole life training your brain for certain kinds of tasks, and then suddenly the job description changes?

Naturally, you try to figure it out the only way you know how. Books. Google. Research.

You spend your nocturnal hours with a baby on one boob and a phone in one hand, trying to figure out the answers.

You are suffering from information overload, and you still aren't finding peace and joy.

Maybe it's time to try a more feminine way of learning?

A Universal Story of Motherhood

This story is told and retold in breastfeeding books and classes and is one of my personal favourites. I even contacted the zoo to check it was true, and it is!

In the 1980s, there was a gorilla in Columbus Zoo in Ohio who was born and raised in captivity. She'd never had any experience of motherhood, she didn't have any friends who were mothers, she'd never even met a baby gorilla before.

She fell pregnant on a breeding program and her healthy baby was born. But she could not breastfeed her baby and it did not end well.

Later, the gorilla fell pregnant again, and this time the zookeepers were paying much closer attention. They decided to invite human mothers from La Leche League to come and breastfeed in front of her enclosure.

The volunteers sat there regularly throughout her pregnancy, breastfeeding their babies, and the gorilla showed more interest as her pregnancy progressed.

But when her baby was born, she still wasn't entirely sure what to do. The zookeepers quickly called the volunteers again and they came and sat right where the gorilla could see. This time the gorilla watched closely.

A human mother picked up her baby, cradled him to her chest, offered her breast and the baby fed. The gorilla mother mimicked her. She picked up her baby, cradled him to her chest, offered her breast and the baby fed.

A New Paradigm

Notice there were no charts or statistics or diagrams. No routines or interventions. There was no equipment.

Time and time again, I see women who want to breastfeed being overloaded with task-oriented, mathematical and rational solutions. Mothers are shown photos of 'correct latch', read books full of conflicting information and are shown videos of swallowing and sucking. We are told to go on special diets and weigh our babies and express milk at specific times of day and measure millilitres of milk and time feeds and count wet nappies...

Confused and overwhelmed yet?

It seems to me that the more we *know* about breastfeeding, the harder it is to actually breastfeed.

This is because breastfeeding, like all mothering skills, is something we learn by feeling and doing. And it's something we learn together, with support from other mothers.

And today, sometimes it feels, just like that gorilla, that we are mothering in captivity.

We all know that it takes a village to raise a child. In lieu of a village, we get lost in the expert advice quagmire.

23

Intuition

One of the classic pieces of advice you have probably received as a mother, especially in the face of this information frenzy, is to trust your intuition.

It sounds so simple, but when people first gave me this advice as a brand new mother, I remember having no idea what it actually meant. Intuition seemed like a fantasy and totally out of reach for me. Sometimes there's so much outside noise interfering with your ability to tune in to your intuition that it's difficult to know where to start.

Luckily, there is a really simple way to combat this onslaught of advice.

Intuition is simply a thinking process. It is the ability to make a quick, automatic decision without a lot of conscious thought.[1]

You know that feeling when you drive home and once you get there you realise that you can't remember any of it? You don't know if the lights were red, or if you put your indicator on, or if you stopped at the zebra crossing. But somehow, on autopilot, you got home safely.

You performed that task without cognitive thinking or conscious effort because you've done it a hundred times before.

Intuition is not a message from the universe or magical thinking. It's simply a state of being so experienced at something that you can read the situation rapidly and make a decision without much work.

This is because your brain has switched into autopilot by moving the task from a 'thinking' task to an 'intuitive' task.

When you've only had your baby for a week, you haven't had time to get to know your baby's cries or body language. You're not yet sure what it looks like when your baby is tired.

When you're told to use your intuition but you don't yet have a reservoir of experience to draw on, you draw a blank.

Next time someone tells you to listen to your intuition, what they really mean is 'practice makes perfect'.

Well, nothing's perfect. But you definitely need practice! And here's how.

The Magic of Mistakes

You might feel like there is something wrong with you because there is an expectation that mothering is an innate ability, one you seem to be lacking.

The cult of the instant, omniscient mother does not allow for the true messiness of real-life learning.

Generally, when you learn a new skill like playing an instrument or speaking a language, you expect to make mistakes along the way.

And when you learn to breastfeed or settle your baby to sleep or soothe his crying, you will make mistakes too.

And that's okay, because you're learning. And your brain is primed for learning right now.

Mistakes are not the problem. They are the solution.

Naomi Stadlen wrote one of my favourite mothering books, *What Mothers Do — Especially When It Looks Like Nothing*. In it, she explains beautifully the value of mistakes.

"If she feels disorientated, this is not a problem requiring bookshelves of literature to put right. No, it is exactly the right state of mind for the teach-yourself process that lies ahead of her.

A mother needs to feel safe enough to risk feeling uncertain. People who offer advice cannot know all the details of her situation. They also don't usually have to live with the long-term consequences of their advice. A mother needs time to 'grow' into parenthood, together with her partner. She needs enough confidence to experiment and change her mind a few times. She needs to learn that some of her ideas work. The most uncertain and under-confident beginner can gradually turn herself into a unique mother.

The miracle is that mothers manage to survive at all in such an expert-ridden climate. After lonely periods of confusion, they suddenly discover that they are starting to understand their babies. As their babies grow, so does their confidence."
— Naomi Stadlen

Intuition may not be magical, but there's magic in making mistakes.

Feeling Out of Control

Making mistakes is difficult, sometimes nearly impossible, for many new mothers, which is one of the reasons we so often turn to experts.

Many women, prior to actually being a mother, plan to be an easy-going mother. When the reality hits though, the very thought of making a single tiny mistake when it comes to your baby can be distressing. Suddenly the stakes are high.

Instead of being serene and unruffled — as they had hoped to be — many mothers find themselves obsessively checking that their baby is breathing, compulsively washing their hands or aggressively defending their baby against visitors.

Rather than being distressed by this unexpected change in character, I believe that it can help to see this as a part of nature's grand plan. A period of maternal preoccupation and hypervigilance would obviously result in a considerably well protected baby.

However, if such feelings are paralysing or out of control, or are interfering with your ability to live the life you want to live, then it's time to have a chat to a professional about your mental health. Your GP, family doctor or primary care provider is always a good starting place and can suggest resources to support you and your baby.

Decluttering Your Brain

It can be discouraging to know that your brain will change and even lose volume when you are pregnant.[2] But rather than seeing all these things as deficits, you can try and picture it as fine-tuning, recalibrating or decluttering.

It's a myth that we only use 10% of our brains; actually your wonderful brain is maxed out doing brilliant things! Evolution isn't wasteful.

Instead, imagine your brain is a filing cabinet. Everything is organised in alphabetical order and in different categories. It's safe and comfortable because you've lived with this filing system for many years. It's packed full of skills and information and all the things you deemed important at some point in your old life.

But when you become a mother, the whole filing cabinet is tipped out to make room for the skills and information that are a priority in your new life. If you want to fit in all the stuff you're going to need to support you in motherhood, you have to figure out what are you going to let go of, which bits no longer serve you.

During this period of decluttering (that stage of neuroplasticity and rapid learning), the breakneck speed of the changes can be overwhelming and exhausting. It can feel messy, disorganised and chaotic. It can go on and on and on.

Over time, your brain will slowly put everything back into the filing cabinet, leaving some stuff out and also adding plenty of new skills and information in. This reorganising means you'll come out the other side with an enriched brain.

Loving

The Calm and Connection Response

So much has been written about the fight or flight response that it's become a household concept, which says something about the focus of our culture. It took a mother to notice that we also have a calm and connection response, and to dedicate her life to studying it.

Kerstin Uvnäs Moberg is a specialist in women's health and female physiology, and has worked within these fields for more than 30 years. She has pioneered research into the biology of women and the extraordinary peptide oxytocin, the so-called 'hormone of love and wellbeing'. As a researcher, she has demonstrated the behavioural, psychological and physiological effects of oxytocin during the key stages in a woman's life; birth, breastfeeding and menopause.[16]

As a mother of four, she found she experienced "a state diametrically opposed" to the pre- motherhood stressors of life; her feelings of "calm and connection" were opposite to those of "challenge, competition and performance".[1]

And this is the second significant way in which your brain changes when you become a mother. Your biology prepares you to fall in love.

What is Oxytocin?

There has been much research into the biological effects of oxytocin in women, and researchers are learning more all the time. Kerstin, who has published more than 400 scientific papers and several books on oxytocin and its effects on the physiology and health of women, describes in her book *The Oxytocin Factor:*[1]

"It's like putting together a puzzle that has some missing pieces; by joining the pieces we do have, we can take a few steps back, see the picture from a larger perspective, and thereby get an idea of how the final calm and connection system is most likely to look."

Oxytocin was originally discovered and isolated from a pregnant cat by pharmacologist and physiologist Sir Henry Dale in 1909. In fact, the hormone is found in every mammal, not just humans and not just women. Nonetheless, at the time, he named it oxytocin, meaning *quick birth* in Latin.

Later on, he discovered that it facilitates the milk ejection reflex, which is also known as *letdown* — not my favourite term! And for many decades the hormone was only known for its starring role in pregnancy, birth and breastfeeding.

More recently, researchers have broadened their horizons and discovered that there are oxytocin receptors not only in the breasts and uterus, but also in the brain, suggesting that the purpose of oxytocin is not simply physical, but also emotional. The effects of oxytocin go beyond purely physical responses, such as causing contractions of your uterus and milk ducts, and extend into the realm of your personality and temperament.[2]

Now the hormone has come into fashion. If there was a popularity contest for hormones, oxytocin would win the decade. And for good reason!

Oxytocin is that sweet, gooey, mushy feeling of falling of love. It's like listening to your favourite music and dancing and losing yourself in the moment. It's singing with friends. Oxytocin is a long, warm hug. It's crying when you watch the news. It's gazing into your baby's eyes and forgetting that the rest of the world exists.

While the word might literally mean *quick birth*, we now know that oxytocin is not just for birth. It's for life. And most of all, for love.

Throughout this section of the book, I rely heavily on breastfeeding research, simply because it is more available and quantifiable than changes in personality and temperament. But, like Kerstin's puzzle, if you delve deeper into the story of oxytocin and breastfeeding, these can be viewed as a symbol for deeper, more psychological changes, even if you don't actually breastfeed.

Falling in Love

There are many ways we can see how oxytocin is designed to help you fall in love, beginning with conception.

Oxytocin is released during orgasm to connect you to your partner so that you stay together in child-raising.[1]

Oxytocin peaks immediately after childbirth to expel the placenta and prevent excessive bleeding. It is the euphoria and love-at-first-sight feeling that some mothers experienced after a healthy, happy birth.

During breastfeeding, the physical act of suckling facilitates oxytocin release and milk ejection. This further strengthens the bond you have with your baby, making you stick around, even during the long and lonely nights.[2]

Beyond Love

The broad-reaching effects of oxytocin in terms of personality and temperament are only just being uncovered and understood. It's possible that oxytocin not only helps you fall in love, but also literally changes the way you experience the world. For the better!

Oxytocin is crucial in regulating childbirth and lactation, giving us some insight into why the emotional experience of these biological functions is so critical to their success.[5]

Here are some examples.

Oxytocin can decrease your sensitivity to stress and pain, thereby assisting during childbirth and in postpartum recovery, growth and healing, and overall wellbeing.[1; 3]

Breastfeeding women can become more social, calmer and more tolerant of monotony and boredom, which is helpful when you are changing your baby's nappy for the 678th time.[6]

Oxytocin plays a role in positive social interactions and bonding.[6; 7] There is extensive published literature showing that good relationships have a positive effect on health, and oxytocin is a contributor to this phenomenon. [7] And having good relationships can assist in reaching out to others, making it more possible for you to find the village you need to support you in your motherhood journey.

Oxytocin has an anti-stress effect, increases your milk supply and can lower blood pressure, which are all good health benefits![6; 8]

Oxytocin increases the speed and sensitivity in reading facial expressions, which is an essential skill for mothering non-verbal infants.[1; 4]

33

In a nutshell, oxytocin can make you healthy, happy and in love with your baby! This extraordinary hormone is designed to help you be the mum you want to be.

Oxytocin is nature's nectar for your peace and joy in motherhood.

Nature's Grand Plan

Maybe you lose track of time and can't remember when your baby last fed or slept. Maybe you feel so much empathy that you can't read the news anymore. Maybe your breasts leak milk everywhere seconds before you even hear your baby wake up! It's all part of the plan.

But what if it's not going to plan?

When Things Don't Go to Plan

There are many factors that can sabotage nature's oxytocin-boosting grand plan.

Some mothers feel stressed, bored or vigilant. They can't sleep even when the baby sleeps. Breastfeeding might feel tense, and they have low milk supply for no apparent reason. They are overly independent, unable to ask for help, or even accept help when it's offered. They may feel judgmental, competitive or controlling.

Maybe you know a mother who feels like this. Maybe you are a mother who feels like this.

Don't despair, next up you will learn how to boost your oxytocin levels naturally and easily, and how to avoid the things that are sabotaging your postpartum peace and joy.

Oxytocin Busters

While oxytocin plays a starring role in pregnancy, birth and breastfeeding, simply having a baby does not guarantee high oxytocin levels. There are many environmental factors that can sabotage nature's grand plan, and they fit broadly under a single category: stress.

Major physical events that are related to oxytocin are easy to measure. For example, research has shown that mothers who give birth by Caesarean section experience fewer oxytocin spikes during breastfeeding.[6]

It is difficult to know which came first, the chicken or the egg, since oxytocin regulates strong contractions and the milk ejection reflex in the first place. Are women struggling with birth and breastfeeding because they are stressed? Or are they stressed because they are struggling with birth and breastfeeding? Without adequate postpartum care, it can become a vicious cycle.

And since we know that there are psychological implications of oxytocin too, it's likely that your emotional experience of the transformation to motherhood is deeply impacted by your stress levels as well.

If you gave birth by Caesarean section or didn't breastfeed, this may all sound like bad news. But in the same way your environment can lower your oxytocin, it can also increase your oxytocin, and it's easy to underestimate the impact of the hundreds of small decisions we make on a daily basis.

Why You Should Sweat the Small Stuff!

Being in an unfamiliar environment may be stressful for you, inhibiting your oxytocin release.[2] Many mothers can relate to having trouble breastfeeding in crowded, noisy, public places, but have you considered the way in which visitors or mess or chores are impacting your feeling of calm, privacy and comfort at home, and therefore your ability to breastfeed even in your own house?

There could be many tiny stressful events sabotaging your oxytocin levels every day.

Are you feeling socially isolated? Or exhausted by chit-chat and entertaining? Do you feel pressured by conflicting advice or too many experts? Has running your household become overwhelming? Have charts or rules or schedules been dominating your life? Do you feel cold or hungry or tired? Are you getting enough rest?

While it's easy to understand the way oxytocin works when you look at major events, try taking a close-up look at your life too. Your oxytocin levels are changing from minute to minute, so there are many subtler stressors in your life that may be raising or reducing your oxytocin levels on a daily basis.

And these smaller points may feel more within your control.

Let's create a plan for boosting your love hormones, starting now.

Oxytocin Boosters

If you feel your oxytocin levels are low, that doesn't necessarily mean that you have a syndrome or deficiency. You don't need injections or nasal sprays. But if you do want some help getting the love hormones flowing, there's plenty to be done.

There are oh-so-many simple things you can do to give yourself an oxytocin boost without any special equipment. The best news? You can do them from home in your pyjamas! Here are just a few examples.

Loving Touch

In a culture that focuses primarily on the wellbeing of babies, you are probably well aware of the benefits of touch for babies through concepts such as kangaroo care, skin-on-skin or baby massage. What is less often discussed is how essential this loving touch is for Newborn Mothers too.

One of the reasons I originally coined the term Newborn Mothers in 2010 was to express the way that a mother is every bit as sensitive and vulnerable as her baby during those early months. Every newborn baby has a Newborn Mother, and you have remarkably similar needs.

One of those needs is for loving touch, such as stroking, massage and hugs, which all act to increase oxytocin. [6; 7]

Newborn babies seem to know this instinctively, as they nuzzle and suckle and even knead you with their tiny fists. But in general, babies need to receive more touch than they are able to give, and many mothers long for a less needy touch from people other than their own children.

37

I remember visiting my doctor after my first baby was born. Having her hands on me — even through my clothes and only for a few minutes — was absolutely heavenly. It felt restorative, grounding and healing, and now I understand why!

Massage is one of my favourite ways of boosting a new mother's oxytocin. That's why in my work as a postpartum doula, I offer a massage to the mothers I work with at every postpartum home visit.

Occasionally mothers feel 'touched out'. If this is the case for you, listen to your body and give yourself some space. Your body, not me or my advice, will tell you the best way to increase your oxytocin levels at any given time.

Comfort Food

Food is more than nutrition; it has the potential to heal us emotionally too. While emotional eating can be problematic in some circumstances, we can't overlook that food intake is related to an increase in oxytocin, allowing us to achieve satisfaction.[2]

Just like touch on your skin, Kerstin Uvnäs Moberg proposes that eating is like an internal massage. When food is moving through your digestive system, it stimulates the vagal nerve, which increases oxytocin. In fact, large amounts of oxytocin are produced inside the gastrointestinal tract.[2]

It's hardly surprising that so many cultures have rituals and ceremonies including food, because we connect more deeply with one another on a full stomach. We'll learn more about specific postpartum food later on.

And you can also breastfeed more easily[7] when you are satisfied from a meal, so keep some snacks by your breastfeeding chair!

Enjoy your food and eat mindfully to maximise the emotional benefits. Food cooked for you will be packed with extra love too!

Warmth

When we talk about warmth, it can imply both a temperature and an emotional state, and that's because applying physical warmth may increase oxytocin and therefore emotional warmth.[2]

We all have experiences of how feeling physically warm and cosy made us also feel relaxed and companionable, like sharing stories around a campfire, or having a cup of hot tea with an old friend.

Like other oxytocin systems, it works something like a circuit. High oxytocin levels increase our body temperatures, and physical warmth increases our oxytocin.

To get yourself on the positive upward spiral of oxytocin, make sure that your home, clothing and company are warm.

Support and Connection

Since oxytocin is so deeply related to bonding, having the right companionship during your transition to motherhood is essential.

It would be easy to assume that *more* support is always better, but in reality, the type of support and the person who gives the support is really the critical factor.

Let's look first at breastfeeding as an example.

Research on the role of mothers' mothers and of partners in supporting breastfeeding is conflicting. In some cases their involvement helps, and in others it doesn't.[10; 11; 12]

A partner's *presence* generally helps the motherhood process, but their practical support sometimes inhibits it. This implies that emotional support is important and valuable for mothers, but interfering with baby care can disrupt many of the biological processes that are intended to unfold during those early weeks.[11]

When it comes to mothers being supported by their own mothers, the biggest indicator of successful support appears to be whether or not the now-grandmother breastfed her own children. A newborn grandmother without lived experience of breastfeeding does not improve breastfeeding outcomes for her daughter, even when she is taught breastfeeding information.[12]

This suggests that it's critical to take a step back from book-based *knowledge*, and allow mothers and babies to simply spend time together, getting to know one another, trusting their natural love hormones to inform their instincts.

This is perhaps why having visitors is often stressful, even when you feel lonely and isolated. In a culture with no framework for how to support Newborn Mothers, visitors often bring inappropriate gifts, expect to be entertained, overstay their welcome and want to hold your baby.

Ideal company for a Newborn Mother would be someone emotionally supportive, who listens to your big feelings without judgment or advice. These visitors would offer practical support that is unrelated to baby care, such as cooking and cleaning.

When it comes to building your village, loving connection is what counts, not information or knowledge.

Rest and Activity

Meditation, prayer, mindfulness, breathing, tai chi, yoga, chanting... different cultures and religions have found different paths to peace and joy. There seems to be some relationship between oxytocin and these calming pursuits, including sleep.

One small study found that oxytocin administration assisted in falling asleep faster, but caused more REM sleep.[13] It makes perfect sense that your brain is programmed to sleep more efficiently, but less deeply, now that you have a baby to care for 24 hours a day. While oxytocin generally promotes sleep, it can also make you more alert. Perhaps you sleep with one eye open now that you have a vulnerable newborn to protect.[2]

In its typical fashion, the way oxytocin works is quite paradoxical, because it is context-dependent, and this is seen clearly in the relationship between meditation and oxytocin.

In his explorations of oxytocin as the 'moral molecule', Paul Zak researched many different religious practices and their effects on oxytocin. His small studies found that singing, dancing and other rituals from many of the world's religions increased oxytocin. But when he came to study meditation, the results were variable.[17]

He visited a Quaker service where they sat for an hour in communal meditation and he found:

"There was no overall change in the average OT [oxytocin]. But this was because roughly half the group had a powerful

41

increase, and the other half had a powerful decrease. It seems that, while sitting in silent contemplation can create a feeling of increased closeness in some, in others it creates the inattention known as boredom. "[17]

Here's another paradox! Exercise also appears to increase oxytocin, one of the reasons we feel so good after a workout.[1]

It appears that the *balance* of rest and activity is what counts, and you'll have to tune in to your body to figure out what you need to do in order to increase your oxytocin levels right now.

How do You Know if it's Working?

There are plenty of things you can do to increase your oxytocin, a long hug, a warm cuppa with a friend, singing a song, taking a nap, having a massage, walking in nature... There are many roads to peace and joy, and which road you choose will depend on your culture, personality, circumstances and preferences.

How will you know if it's working? You'll feel peace and joy!

If you are struggling under the weight of conflicting advice and feeling overwhelmed, the best thing you can do is tune in with how you are feeling.

Do what you love, and your love hormones will flow.

And when your love hormones flow, your milk will flow, your blood pressure will drop, your body will heal, you'll feel less pain, your mental health will improve, and you'll have more tolerance for the monotony of motherhood.

You'll be the happy, healthy mother you always planned to be.

New Extremes of Emotion

Many mothers will know that it's not as simple as having a baby and then feeling blissed out all the time. It's a little more complicated than that.

If you look too closely at the details of oxytocin research, you may find yourself confused.

In her book *Oxytocin: The Biological Guide to Motherhood*[2], Kerstin Uvnäs Moberg writes:

"The effects spectrum that oxytocin induces is context-dependent. The effects of oxytocin are always aimed at protecting the offspring. Therefore, exposure to oxytocin can induce aggression and stress effects under certain conditions necessary to ensure the survival of the offspring."

Put simply, if you feel safe, oxytocin may make you more relaxed and loving, but if you feel threatened, oxytocin may make you more aggressive and defensive. Although oxytocin is generally associated with feelings of peace and calm, it can also make you hypervigilant as you ferociously defend your babies from all sorts of real and perceived threats, such as germs and visitors.[15]

Oxytocin is the reason why your happiness scale was altered, and you feel a heightened sense of emotion.

And since oxytocin triggers appropriate mothering behaviours designed to protect your baby depending on your circumstances, those circumstances are highly important.

43

It's never been more vital to listen to your body and do what you can to create an environment that supports your peace and joy. Because in the right circumstances, oxytocin is designed to make you *and* your baby thrive, not just survive.

Love Conquers All

I'm not a big fan of rules, but there is one rule I always honour. I call it the golden rule.

Love conquers all.

I want you to keep this in mind as a framework whenever you consider new information and make decisions. I want you to ask yourself one simple question.

How does this feel for you?

Find what brings you peace and joy. And do it. Every single day.

Variety

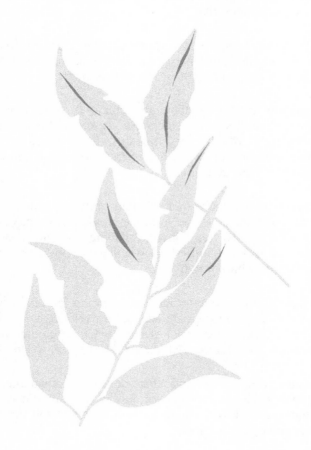

Gender

If you happen to be born with a uterus and breasts, and use them to birth and feed your baby, then you have a biological headstart in the oxytocin race. But much fuss has been made throughout recent history of women's hormones, often as a scapegoat to delegitimise our emotions, concerns and desires, and often to uphold conservative views of what a family should look like.

While researchers are now seeing that there are differences in the brains and hormones of men and women, we still have much more in common than what sets us apart.

Everybody has within them the potential to be feminine or masculine. We all can choose to apply this potential appropriately in different situations. Early parenthood is a clear example of a season where choosing a feminine approach is more relevant.

Everyone has oxytocin: men, women, children, grandparents and non-parents. And you'll notice most of those oxytocin-increasing actions don't involve having or using a uterus at all, and work regardless of whether you are genetically related to the child or not.

Put simply, if you invest your time in caring for a baby, your brain will make appropriate adaptations relating to learning and loving. This makes a lot of sense when considered in the context of *alloparenting*, which we'll be exploring later on.

No matter who you are and what your family looks like, you can unlock the secrets to peace and joy in parenthood with oxytocin, and it will happen naturally when you do what brings you peace and joy.

Newborn Fathers

However… in my 10 years of experience working with new families, I began to notice something unexpected. Sometimes I would visit during those early weeks and find mum curled up in bed, blissing out with her baby. Meanwhile dad was taking a trip to the hardware store or getting a promotion at work that involved longer hours.

It definitely appeared that for some (but not all) fathers, their hormones were reacting differently to their partners' after having a baby.

I found a possible explanation for this in Paul Zak's book *The Moral Molecule*, in which he describes a time he went to his friend Linda's wedding and saw how oxytocin responded during the ceremony. He found something truly remarkable.[1]

"The changes in individual oxytocin levels at Linda's ceremony could be mapped out like the solar system, with the bride as the sun. Between the first and second blood draws, which were only an hour apart, Linda's own level shot up by 28 percent. And for each of the other people tested, the increase in oxytocin was in direct proportion to the likely intensity of emotional engagement in the event. The mother of the bride? Up 24 percent. The father of the groom? Up 19 percent. The groom himself? Up 13 percent… and on down the line with siblings and friends with more peripheral roles to play.

But why, you may ask, would the groom's increase be less than his father's? We'll get into this sort of thing more deeply along the way, but testosterone is one of several other hormones that can interfere with the release of oxytocin. Not too surprising when you think about it, I also found that the groom's testosterone had surged 100 percent!

Our little study at the wedding had demonstrated, on the hoof, just the kind of graded and contingent sensitivity that allows oxytocin to guide us between trust and wariness, generosity and self-protection, not only in response to the official nature of relationships — my mother, my son-in-law, my dreaded classmate, a complete stranger — but in response to social cues in the moment. " — Paul Zak

In other words, it's possible our hormones have the ability to read a social situation and adjust in order for us to step into the appropriate role in a team. The point here is to not measure the exact hormones, but to understand that humans are both social and biological creatures. We are designed to work in teams, in synchronicity.

In fact, research has shown that there is co-ordination or synchrony of the brain responses of both parents to their baby's cues.[2] Such studies shed light on the brain's basis for the profound attachment that occurs during human parenting.

We are going to take a deeper look at the history and evolution of families very soon, but for now imagine a cave mum gazing into her baby's eyes. She is getting warm and cuddly social cues, which draw her more deeply into her nurturing role. Meanwhile, in order to support his vulnerable new family, cave dad steps into his protector and provider role. He wants to make sure they are sheltered and fed, and that there are no sabre-tooth tigers at the door.

Both roles are beautiful and essential and valuable, and in those early weeks, it makes sense that they are allocated according to whichever parent happened to give birth physically. Beyond that, you can apply what you've learned so far to transcending these traditional gender roles, if you wish.

Roles and Responsibilities

While a birthing parent might have a biological headstart, what often keeps them in the role of primary caregiver is in fact cultural.

It usually begins as a small divergence of roles, often a practical decision based on whose body is providing the milk for the baby. After many months and years of experience, it becomes a gaping chasm as one parent is vastly more confident and capable than the other, simply because they've had more time on the job.

Where this becomes problematic is where roles are divided along gender lines, without any thought for the preferences and skills of each parent. At its worst, it can reinforce the gender stereotypes of the incompetent dad and the superwoman mum, and in the long-run it can contribute to women doing the lion's share of domestic work, including emotional labour like remembering birthdays and volunteering in the classroom.

If traditional roles are working in your family, then there is no reason to change. However, if the roles you find yourselves in are not making you happy, there is no need to feel trapped.

Throughout the time I've been writing this book, I have still been breastfeeding my youngest child. At this very moment, my husband is at home with our three small children helping our daughter enter a cake baking and decorating competition and I'm at a hotel writing a book; our financial contributions to the family are equal.

Once those gendered roles of the early months have served their purpose, there is no reason to stick with them, unless you want to. If you prefer, you can transcend those roles simply by applying what you've learned so far.

49

The more opportunities any parent has for hands-on learning and the more freedom they have to learn by trial and error, the more their skills and confidence grow.

And the more time any parent or caregiver spends with a child, the more oxytocin they experience. This oxytocin bonds us to our children and helps us enjoy parenting, so that we want to do more of it.

Have a chat with your partner about the different stages, seasons and roles in your family. If and when you are ready, you'll need to step out of the way, so your partner can have a chance to rewire their brain too.

The Future

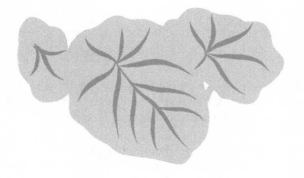

Upgrading Your Operating System

A friend of mine is studying law and also happens to have two children. She recently got a distinction in her law assignment, then couldn't remember where she had parked her car...

I know exactly how frustrating baby brain is!

Think of it like upgrading the operating system for your brain. It can take a while to find your way around, and it's kind of annoying not knowing where anything is anymore. But in the long run, the new features are worth the steep learning curve.

So what exactly do you stand to gain from this enrichment program or 'system upgrade'?

Long-Term Benefits

While *Newborn Mothers* focusses on postpartum, the immediate months and years after giving birth, there are also many longer-term benefits of becoming a mother.

Katherine Ellison wrote a brilliant book called *The Mommy Brain: How Motherhood Makes Us Smarter*, inspired by her own experiences of becoming a mother.[1]

She delayed having children for many years, as she had been repeatedly told she would lose her brain when she had a baby and didn't wanted to jeopardise her successful career as an investigative reporter. When she finally had children, her experience was different from what she had expected.

"I didn't feel particularly damaged, after all. True, I was complaining a lot more, but I was also accomplishing a lot more. Though I often felt frazzled, I was more motivated, excited by what I was learning at work and at home...

Although I'd had newspaper deadlines before, never had I faced the unparalleled urgency of a baby who needed to breastfeed, or a preschool teacher at the close of day, both of which taught me a new kind of focus.

Within two years of our move to California, despite constant interruptions, I had finished my book, gone on a speaking tour, launched a freelance career, helped my kids adjust to a new community, supervised repairs to our home, found a great circle of friends and tracked down a qualified expert to help a babysitter afflicted with early-stage leprosy. I had many more reasons for worry, yet, to my surprise, I felt calmer. And I kept running into other mothers who felt the same way." — Katherine Ellison

She had uncovered a largely untold scientific story and went on to develop the hopeful idea that motherhood makes us smarter. Through her research and interviews, she found five positive attributes of a 'baby-boosted brain'.

The first is your senses. You probably experienced super smelling power during pregnancy but perhaps didn't realise that there are longer-term and broader improvements to your perception, including more sensitivity to sight, sound and touch.

The second positive change relates to efficiency. I'll bet you can achieve remarkable feats while your baby takes a 45-minute nap. It's a miracle we get anything done at all with no sleep and constant interruptions, yet we do!

Third, you become more resilient. Oxytocin can act as a buffer to stress. The tend-and-befriend response is a more feminine alternative to fight-or-flight, and the way we rally together as mothers is a huge source of strength.

Fourth, you become more ambitious and motivated. Having children gives you a greater sense of urgency and a stronger desire to create a better future. Certainly, my own experience of becoming a mother makes me determined to create better opportunities for my daughter and be a role model.

And finally, mothers are more emotionally intelligent. You are better at reading social cues, resolving conflict and restraining yourself when all you really want to do is yell, swear, and get in a car and drive… anywhere. Even though your children may push all your buttons, you're still here, right?

Katherine Ellison argues, quite convincingly, that motherhood makes our brains not only better at motherhood, but better at life in general. For example, mothers make excellent employees, politicians and leaders, not in spite of having babies, but because of it!

Be kind to yourself as your brain is busy rewiring. It's worth the wait.

Your Village

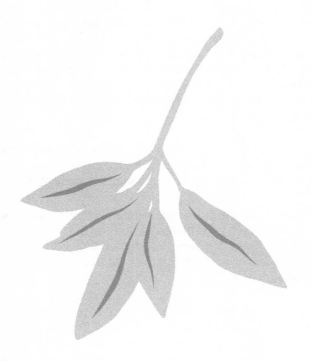

Big Brain, Small Pelvis

Have you ever noticed how human babies are vulnerable compared with other species? Our babies can't walk, talk or feed themselves and they rely on adults to care intensively for them for many, many years. Extended childhood may not seem like a particularly effective survival strategy, but what if it is?

If you've ever wondered why human babies are born so vulnerable, you have probably heard of the obstetric dilemma. This is the theory that newborn humans are born prematurely, before their brains grow too big to fit through a woman's upright pelvis. That is; our ancestors had to make evolutionary compromises, and in walking upright, our pelvic size was contained for locomotive efficiency; therefore, our babies had to be born earlier, before they can walk, talk or feed themselves.

Since it was first proposed in the 1950s or thereabouts, this has been the common explanation for vulnerable babies and risky birth in medicine, biology, anatomy and anthropology.

Dr Holly Dunsworth, an anthropologist and — you guessed it — a mother, tested the obstetric dilemma hypothesis. She and her colleagues compared human and primate neonatal brain size and gestation length to find out if our babies are indeed born early:[2]

"Compared to other primates, humans actually gestate as long as or a little longer than expected for a mother's body size. Our neonates are as large as or larger than expected, and so are their brains. We may have only a third of our adult brain size at birth, but we are born with the largest newborn brain of all primates. Our newborn brain size is only relatively smaller than a chimp newborn's because

56

the denominator, adult brain size, is three times greater in humans than in chimpanzees. So we may have more brain to grow after we're born than a chimpanzee does, but that isn't a strong case for describing us as being born 'early'." — Dr Holly Dunsworth

They also drew on studies of the mechanics and energetics of human walking and running to test the idea that wider hips (women) were less efficient at movement than slimmer hips (men). Is it true that bipedal inefficiency is what has constrained our pelvis size and caused our babies to be born at a particular time?

"The majority have found no difference, with some finding that females are more economical" and "there is little evidence that pelvic constraints have altered the timing of birth."— Dr Holly Dunsworth[3]

In other words, the assumption that a woman's hips are too small to birth her own baby at the optimal time tells us more about the masculine culture that has been dominating science than it does about childbirth itself.

The most likely reason for the timing of human birth is that the baby's metabolic needs grow beyond what the mother can accommodate. And there's another way of looking at it too.

Perhaps the most interesting thing about disproving the obstetric hypothesis is it frees us up to look at the timing of childbirth from a more social and cultural point of view.

So Holly Dunsworth reframed the question:

"Inventors, artists, and scientists are the usual suspects for symbolising and celebrating the brainy human primate.

However, what if babies, mothers and other caregivers were the real stars in the story of human intelligence? "[1]

What if our babies are not born early at all? What if the timing is perfectly designed? From this new perspective, we can begin to explore what benefits there might be to the human species of being born at that specific stage of development.

I was so excited by this idea that I emailed Holly Dunsworth for clarification. Here is her reply:

"I definitely think it's the journey that's more important than the destination, so what goes into brain development and what goes on during it is the key factor in our evolutionary history more than the resulting huge brain at the end of the process. Our bodies are not broken. There is no obstetrical dilemma!"

What does all this mean?

Well, what if, instead of assuming women's bodies are faulty, we view human babies as being hardwired to experience their brain development in a highly social environment? We've already seen that brains develop differently in different environments; maybe human birth is perfectly timed to give our brains the opportunity to develop in an enriched environment?

When a baby's brain is developing in a womb, it's quiet and dark. The temperature is regulated and there is very little stimulation. After that baby is born, there are lots of cuddles and kisses, there's touch, singing, talking, and rocking. Perhaps this abundance of love and connection during these formative years is what sets our brains on the evolutionary path to becoming the spectacularly smart and caring humans we are today. Maybe it's not that you have a short gestation, or an inadequate pelvis, but that in addition to pregnancy, your baby experiences a stage of social gestation.

If this is in fact the case, it is a brilliant reproductive strategy, one that results in our ultimate success as a species, in intelligent and compassionate people. It requires the generous investment of human mothers and other caregivers over many years and over many generations.

Let's take a look at where it all began in history or *herstory*.

Or quite simply the origins of motherhood.

History

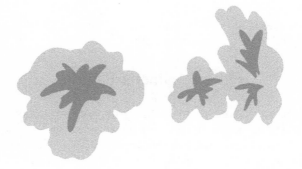

It Takes a Village

About 1.8 million years ago, some highly social apes somewhere on the African continent began to share the care of their babies. This may seem like a barely significant thing, but it's possible that this tiny act set us on the evolutionary path to becoming the empathetic, brainy humans we are today.

This shared care is called *alloparenting* or *cooperative breeding*. Some animals are incredibly protective of their young, but humans will quite happily hand their baby to other humans, because we've learnt to trust each other.

It is this *alloparenting* that affords our babies the opportunity to be born so early in their brain development, and requiring such a huge investment from caregivers.

Given our babies are born so vulnerable, it was never designed to be a one-woman job.

Hunter-Gatherer Families

I want to make it clear that I'm not romanticising or idealising ancient cultures, but it's interesting and useful to look at where we have come from, and the situations and environments our brains and bodies have evolved to expect, over tens of thousands of years.

A hunter-gatherer mother was generally surrounded by her extended family. Just like those apes we've evolved from, we have babies that are highly dependent on a great number of adults. In hunter-gatherer communities, babies were seen as a social responsibility not an individual choice.

Sarah Blaffer Hrdy is an anthropologist, primatologist and author, and of course, a mother of three. She found:

"In groups such as the Efe and Aka Pygmies of central Africa, allomothers actually hold children and carry them about. In these tight-knit communities of communal foragers—within which men, women, and children still hunt with nets, much as humans are thought to have done tens of thousands of years ago—siblings, aunts, uncles, fathers, and grandmothers hold newborns on the first day of life. When University of New Mexico anthropologist Paula Ivey asked an Efe woman, "Who cares for babies?" the immediate answer was, "We all do!" By three weeks of age, the babies are in contact with allomothers 40 percent of the time. By eighteen weeks, infants actually spend more time with allomothers than with their gestational mothers. On average, Efe babies have fourteen different caretakers, most of whom are close kin. According to Washington State University anthropologist Barry Hewlett, Aka babies are within arm's reach of their fathers for more than half of every day."[1]

This may seem exotic compared to nuclear families, but in fact it is the norm throughout human history. The concept of nuclear families with one mum nurturing and one dad providing is really quite bizarre when you see the bigger picture.

Losing the Village

For millions of years — literally — it has taken a village to raise a child. How did we lose our villages? Here's what I believe happened.

Around 200 years ago, industrialisation and colonisation reorganised families. It's been perhaps the most rapid and all-encompassing period of change in the history of human cultures.

63

Now people move to other cities, or even to other countries in order to find work. We live away from extended family and nuclear families have become the norm.

Not only do we mother physically alone, but we have also lost touch with the wisdom of our own mothers and grandmothers. We no longer have access to our elders and we've lost our cultural framework for supporting new families.

And yet, we still need to learn mothering skills, so where do we now turn?

Around 1900, science and medicine were gaining popularity, and they began to encroach on oral history and what were traditionally more feminine areas of knowledge, including childbirth and breastfeeding. For the first time, there was a large number of experts, most of whom were not women, and sometimes not even parents themselves. This has led to the commodification of motherhood and sabotaged breastfeeding by placing the knowledge outside the mother in the hands of so-called specialists.

While the Industrial Revolution undoubtedly improved our quality of life in many ways, it also changed the way we think about things like efficiency and productivity. Not only were our family structures changed, but also our values and these values were reflected in the parenting beliefs of the time. Rigid schedules and routines came into fashion, and mothers were told to restrict cuddling their baby to only 10 minutes a day, and to breastfeed only once every four hours. Mechanical processes became popular both in industry and in more human realms, as though data has the answer to why your baby won't sleep or why you are having trouble breastfeeding.

And since productivity and efficiency are still desirable in a masculine culture, many of these attitudes persist today.

This being said, these parenting trends rarely happen top-down, experts don't rise to popularity in a vacuum. These rigid parenting recommendations were likely welcomed by many mothers at that time, as a very natural reaction to the situation that they found themselves in. Mothers were all alone and no longer able to mother so intensively as they had done when that care was shared by the whole family unit. It follows that mothers were relieved when they were told that it was okay to stop parenting to the extent it was done previously.

Naturally, many babies failed to thrive.

In the 1970s, along came attachment theory, and this was a really important time for babies. We discovered a baby's needs for nurture and we understood that emotional investment was crucial for baby's immediate survival, as well as long-term health and happiness.

But attachment science developed in extremely unusual human circumstances, "based on a (probably idealized) model of middle-class Anglo-American family life in the 1950s that does not correspond to the circumstances of care for most of the world's babies."[2]

Responsive parenting was great news for babies, but not so great news for mums, because now mums were being expected to do the job of raising children alone, and provide all that nurturing themselves, when traditionally it had been shared by alloparents.

As mothers, we are programmed to make many sacrifices for our children, so our babies in general are thriving again. But it is little wonder that mothers nowadays feel exhausted and overwhelmed by the enormous role that was once shared by their whole village.

65

Now it's time for us to reconnect with what Newborn Mothers need and develop our social responsibility for families so that you can be healthy and happy too.

What Mothers Need

I don't expect you'll want to hand your newborn around to 14 different people every day! You might not even know that many people who you'd trust with your baby, but you still need a village.

While transformation is intrinsically intense, it doesn't necessarily have to involve suffering. That suffering is replaced with rewarding and satisfying hard work when we do it with the right support.

Today's village looks different, but it still fulfils your emotional and physical needs as a Newborn Mother.

You Need Emotional Support

We are social creatures, but motherhood today can be desperately lonely and isolating. In order to survive the storm, you need friendships.

Other mothers are on the same journey as you right now. They can provide the companionship you are looking for. They can normalise your experience and what to expect from your baby. Travelling together is less dark and lonely and together, we can figure this out. More experienced mothers are especially valuable for mentoring and guidance, and give us the opportunity to learn in a more feminine way, through observation and immersion.

What other mothers can't always provide is the practical support you need.

There is an extraordinary amount of work required to raise a child. And while it's fun to play with your children, they also need to eat, every single day. And they make crazy amounts of mess. And it's so annoying how they keep growing out of their clothes! Cooking, cleaning and shopping all take vast quantities of time beyond your primary role of caring for your children.

If you are overwhelmed and exhausted by all this work, chances are so are the other women in your mums group. Occasionally you can find ways to support each other; for example, it takes very little extra time to cook a double batch of dinner and give some to another mother. But in general mothers simply don't have the bandwidth to help each other out with shopping, cooking and cleaning, since we all need help with the very same thing.

So we must continue to grow our village beyond other mothers.

You Need Practical Support

We often forget to include men in our village-building efforts. Starting with fathers.

Since parenting is a learned skill, a gap can develop if he is not there during the massive learning curve of the first few months. Like a fork in the road, you suddenly realise that you, the mother, have developed a vast repertoire of domestic skills while his day-to-day life has largely continued on as before.

Often, what it takes for him to step up is for you to step back. Give him time alone with his children to make all the mistakes you have already made, and learn to be the father he wants to be.

67

Grandparents, neighbours, teenagers… anyone can be part of your village. Often the hardest part is reaching out, when this is not the norm in our culture. Asking for help is like flexing a muscle; it gets easier every time you do it.

It's a great idea to buy a part of your village too! Childcare, cleaners and meal delivery services can be an excellent investment in your mental health, and free up your time and energy to be the mum you want to be.

Village Building Today

Now that you understand you need a village, I'm going to teach you exactly how to build yours. It's really easy, all you have to do is…

Ask for help.

I can see you squirming from here, but it's totally worth it!

Here are some experiences of Newborn Mothers I have worked with:

"I spent the first few years of motherhood trying to juggle all the balls! Plus, the constant worry about not earning enough to warrant getting help or support. I learnt the hard way by burning out. It's not easy and I know I struggle with letting go of the control but it feels so good to get help!! Now I would sell my shoes just to have someone come and clean my house every week or so. Asking for help has truly kept me going. I just wish I'd understood how beneficial it would be years ago!!" — Jojo

"I found it hard accepting help when the rest of society looks like they're doing it all on their own (even though they're not). I was almost embarrassed to tell friends about the

help I had because it's not the norm and they'd think I was being indulgent. I found that when I ask for help, people are delighted to be able to give it!" — Lynn

"After giving birth to twins, the maternal health nurse asked me if I needed help at home as I had two older boys as well! I stupidly said, "Oh no, we'll be fine!" I struggled every morning to get everyone dressed and out the door to school until a neighbour said she would do the school run... and bless that woman she did a whole school term!!!! It was such a simple gesture but it made an enormous difference to my day. Although I didn't ask for the help, I did accept it and that was a huge hurdle for me." — Anne-Maree

Asking for Help

As women, we are conditioned to never be too bold, too bossy or too loud. We must not take up too much space, be too angry or too demanding. The patriarchy depends on your compliance.

It's likely there are many cultural expectations that you have internalised and that are preventing you from asking for help. Maybe you are worried about being a burden, or scared of losing control. Perhaps you don't want people to think you are weak, or appear an incompetent mother. You might feel guilty or selfish or ashamed.

In fact, it's normal to get help with things like childcare, cleaning, shopping and cooking. Providing the millions of calories that it takes to raise a human baby to adulthood was never designed to be a one-woman job.

But where to even start!?

By embracing your mother archetype.

69

No-one is the perfect mother, and no-one ever was. It's more helpful to work to your strengths and fill in the gaps with your village.

Maybe you love cleaning and can't relax till the dishes are done, or maybe your house is verging on unhygienic because you prefer to play with your kids.

Maybe you are fastidiously organised, or always running fashionably late.

Maybe you are consistent and predictable, or maybe you're intuitive and emotional. Maybe you prioritise fun, or maybe you prioritise education.

The thing is there's no one correct way to be a mother. Embracing your strengths and outsourcing the rest frees you to be the mum you want to be, and your village will fill in the gaps. Your child will not be deprived!

Face your fears and ask for help. As you build your village, you are playing your part in changing the social norms, and ensuring that future mothers will have access to the village we all so desperately need as well.

Stories

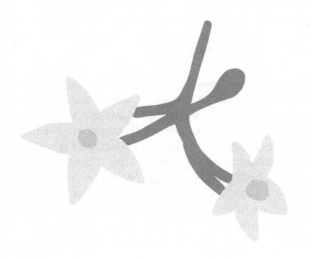

The Wisdom of Elders

Many pregnant women spend their time preparing for birth, but don't have the necessary resources or support they need after the baby arrives. Without the emotional, social and even spiritual support we need, the vast majority of Newborn Mothers feel exhausted, isolated and overwhelmed.

I know there is a different way of experiencing the transition to motherhood.

With a little preparation and a lot of help, the first six weeks after your baby is born — though intense and vulnerable — could also be the best weeks of your life. I know this, because it has been the experience of many of the women I've worked with at this time in their lives.

"Julia gave me permission to bask in the beauty of early motherhood. I didn't touch the housework and I kept the flow of eager visitors to a manageable few. Do you want to know what I did do? I held my baby, I breastfed my baby, I spoke to my new daughter and I told her how much I loved her. Those first few weeks were incredible. Sure, I was tired and I had blistered nipples. And although I felt so emotionally raw and vulnerable I could feel the waves of oxytocin engulfing me. I have never loved so hard or felt so loved in return. It was an intense time. I only wish that every new mother had the ability to feel as protected and nurtured as I did." — Tania

"Working with Julia has allowed me to listen to my body and my whole family benefits. I feel stronger and more capable now with three children than I ever did with two, or even one. I know that it is because I nourished myself during what I now know to be a sacred window of time. I think working with Julia benefited my entire family as well as my relationships. I found that by having explained to relatives that I would be taking six weeks of confinement and the reasons behind it,

72

people were more respectful of my need to rest and therefore relationships were preserved! My husband is a huge fan. I think we both wish that we had Julia's support for our first and second babies! I can honestly say the six weeks after the birth of James were the calmest, most restful and nourishing weeks of my life to date. The experience was so wonderful that many days I even consider that I might like a fourth child... just to experience that blissful love and calm again!"
— Gina

So what's the secret? What are these mothers doing differently from the vast majority of mothers today who feel exhausted, isolated and overwhelmed?

Of course, they are harnessing the power of baby brain by embracing the magic of making mistakes and tuning in to what brings them peace and joy. They are building their villages and asking for help.

And there is one more piece of the puzzle I am about to share with you...

Anthropologists have identified a range of social structures that are designed to protect and support Newborn Mothers, and they've found these same patterns occurring in hundreds of cultures right around the world.

It seems that here in the industrialised world, we've forgotten all about these ancient traditions. When we lost our villages, we also lost touch with the wisdom of our elders.

It's time for a renaissance in the care of our Newborn Mothers.

Theresa — England and Australia

Theresa Clifford was my own mother's midwife when I was born, so it was extra special to have the opportunity to invite her to share her knowledge of postpartum traditions. Theresa was born and raised in the north-east of England and became a midwife simply because it would give her the opportunity to travel.

But she also has midwifery in her family: her grandmother and her grandmother's sisters were known as 'handywomen'.

They were called the handywomen, and they did births, and laying out the dead. I don't remember her telling me because I was quite young when my grandma died. But I remember her daughters telling me, when I first started midwifery, that they used to go with her to the births because they had to bring the sheets home and do the washing. And the daughters had to cook soup, and take soup around to the houses of the people who'd had the babies. Chicken soup is for when you're sick, your immunity is down, when you need to be built up. So that was my little connection to midwifery, a family connection.

The handywomen delivered the baby. Afterwards, they went in and out for days to wash the sheets and to look after the mums, because mums stayed in bed for three days. Even when I first started my training, you stayed in bed for three days. You didn't get out of bed. They weren't allowed up, even to the toilet, I don't think. You'd spend seven to ten days in hospital, and you certainly didn't wash your hair in the first week.

And it was your community that looked after you. Certainly in England, it depended on which social class you were in. Particularly when I was on the district [nursing rounds], we would go round to do antenatal visits. You'd knock on the door, and the woman next door would pop her head out and say, "Oh, she's not there. She's down the road. She's down at number 16." And you'd go down to number 16, and there's eight or ten women sitting around the table, laughing, talking, snotty-nosed kids running around, nappies hanging off them. But they were totally, totally there for each other, and supported each other.

And then you'd go to the other end of town. You'd knock on the door, and you'd see the curtain go, and you'd think, "Oh right, okay, what's gonna happen here?" And she comes to the door with the full make-up, the lipstick on, and the smile on her face. And you'd think, "Ah, this woman's got postnatal depression, I can see it."

When I first started working here in Australia, as a home-birth midwife, I used to insist that the mums got a food roster. And they'd say, "Oh, I can't do that." And I'd say, "Oh, I can't be your midwife then. You need to tell a friend that the midwife told you to get a food roster and for the friend to organise it for you. Give your friend six people that will probably go on it. Let your friend organise it. And they'll do it and you will get a meal every second day for two weeks."

They'd say, "Ah, but he can cook." And I'd say, "I know he can cook, and he can wash, and he can clean, but it's gonna take two of you until 2pm just to sort out this 8lbs of baby. And if there are other kids involved, then his role is more to be with them, while you sleep and feed the baby, and the women bring in the food."

It used to just happen in the community. They looked out for each other. I remember I was at school when my youngest brother was born, and people used to pick us up from school and take us to their house and give us dinner, and then bath us, and take us home in our jammies when the new baby came. So you were just taken in by somebody else and taken home by 5.30pm. There was still family time, but there was nothing for mum to do. She didn't have to cook, she didn't have to bath the kids. She just had to lay clothes out for the next day. We just walked ourselves to school, and after school, you walked back to somebody's house and that's where you got your dinner that night.

We used to bind all the mums' bellies. We used to bind the babies' bellies as well. We used to clean them and bind them, until the cord dropped off. Back then a lot of the women didn't breastfeed, so the ones that didn't breastfeed used to get their breasts bound too. And it was just like a corset thing... Or we might have used old sheets, and just put big safety pins down and tuck their bellies in.

It was for support. It was maybe to help with involution of the uterus, but it was standard that we did belly binding.

At one hospital I worked in, they just threw out the placentas in a waste disposal. In another place, they used to take away the cut membranes, and the membranes used to go to Great Ormond Street Hospital for burn dressings. And in another hospital, they used to go to one of those make-up companies, maybe Elizabeth Arden, for collagen creams and so on.

When I first started doing home-births in Australia, which was 38-39 years ago, by law you had to dispose of the placenta properly. And so it was burnt or buried. With my first clients, I used to always buy them a tree, and so the placenta was placed on the placenta tree.

Placenta encapsulation is new, only in the last eight or ten years. I can remember a woman asking me about placenta encapsulation and I said I didn't know much about it.

Early on, when I was doing my births here, there were always women who would want to eat their placentas. This was 30-40 years ago. We'd just shave a little bit off, little fingernail-

size pieces on some foil, and wrap it up and put it in the freezer. They'd just take one piece and swallow it.

The only ritual I remember for after the birth was a Catholic ritual, which I recall from when my mum had her last baby, when I was nine or ten. I remember her not being able to go out until she'd been churched. She had to go to church to be blessed, not the christening of the baby, but for her to be blessed by the priest. And then there was a baptism of the baby maybe later. She wasn't allowed to resume normal duties or anything until she'd been churched.

Kerry-Ann, Dorothy and Margaret — Nyungar

I live by the Swan River in Western Australia, which is the traditional country of the Nyungar people, one of the oldest living cultures in the world. The Swan River is a natural harbour and white settlement around the area was rapid and dense. The lives of the Nyungar people were devastated, and their language and culture disrupted.

I asked my old neighbour Kerry-Ann Winmar if she could share some of her stories and postpartum knowledge. She invited two more elders to join us. Dorothy Winmar is a Ballardong, Whadjuk and Wagyl Kaip woman with four children and ten grandchildren. Margaret Taylor is a Ballardong and Wagyl Kaip woman who raised seven children of her own plus many foster children and has twenty-nine grandchildren and five great grandchildren. Kerry-Ann herself is a Ballardong, Whadjuk and Wagyl Kaip woman with four children and ten grandchildren. Here are some of their experiences with gwinyart, newborn babies.

Margaret

In the old days, my grandmother took a hold of me and I lived with her forever. It was traditional for the grandparents to take the first born.

Kerry-Ann

When I had my first-born son, my mum and dad took him straight away, so I used to just go and visit my son. He's very close to my mum and dad. It was tradition, my dad used to say, "We get to take the first born baby".

Dorothy

But back in the days, all of the families more or less lived together, so we're all still in that one group.

Margaret

And whoever's got the milk feeds the baby. As long as they got a clean titty and good milk there, just share it around. Say for instance, if I was busy making a damper (munjarly) and Dorothy was there, she'll say, "I'll feed it."

Kerry-Ann

And my mother, grandmother and great-grandmother had to be very strong, because they had inadequate housing. They lived in humpies and tin sheds. They would have bags that would just hang at the front to block out the wind and all that.

I assume that Aboriginal people before colonisation had ways of looking after their babies. I think they would have used kangaroo skins at that time because that was something waterproof so they never got too cold or too wet because the water would trickle off.

Some of our grandmothers could go to the hospital, but they weren't allowed to have the babies inside the hospital — they had to be on the veranda outside where it had a big canvas sheet in it.

I'm very supportive with my own children, moral support, just being there, because now when the baby is born, the mum only stays in hospital for one day. When I had a baby, I had to stay in hospital for a week or two because it was just that period where you had to rest.

Dorothy

Yeah, and they get sent home from hospital too quick these days. The mother's just dropping the baby, then they're coming home. I don't like it anyway, because I'd like the mothers to stay longer to have that bond with that baby.

Kerry-Ann

I think hospitals and midwives are trying to learn a lot more about how to support us and all that, but Aboriginal people, we don't gel with it, because it's too legalistic. It's too many boxes to tick and all that kind of thing. Too much reading, too much talking.

When we support our own family, it's like eye contact, nurturing, just having an elder mother or grandmother, or great-grandmother there. You can feel that love and the encouragement, because it's the way we do things. And it's how we look, how we hold our postures, our eye contact, our body language and all those kinds of things.

79

Margaret

A lot of our babies were born at home and we had our own midwives. They didn't have these degrees; they just knew how to deliver these babies. Because it was something that was always there from the very first beginning.

But I'd never seen a mum being nurtured when they have their babies. They had to make them diapers and cook them feeds. The man would go to work because he couldn't stop working in the welfare days, they were taking kids all the time. So if your kids weren't looked after then... yeah, it was really hard.

The placenta played an important part in Aboriginal significance when babies were born, but unfortunately, when colonisation happened and hospitals happened, they took the placenta away. A lot of the mums were very grieved about that because that was their baby's birthright.

A lot of people, traditional people from remote areas, they always come down and ask if they can take their placenta back. It was a bit of a rift with the health department. When they have the baby, they're happy, but they're sad too because their birthright's taken away. That placenta is their rights to that country. When that baby was born on the reserves or community, they'd bury that placenta there, not far from where the baby was born and that was a ceremonial thing. It was to identify this baby with his homelands; that he's connected to that land, as far as the eyes can see.

Kerry-Ann

And they'd have certain bush foods, like yams and berries and quandongs and all those kinds of things. New mums ate certain parts, the good parts, even the good part of the goanna (bungarra). They ate the tail, the best part, because

80

the tail from down there had all the meat on it. Anything bush, but we encourage them not to have too much takeaway. One kangaroo (yonger) will feed three or four different families. They'd catch the kangaroo. And if there's a widow or woman had a new baby, they would give them the best part of the kangaroo. They would have fed a new mum kangaroo stew, but if they were feeling a bit weak, they would have some of the family members go and get a goanna or an echidna (ningarn) or an emu (waitch). Emu was good because it is high in protein and gives them good balance when their body was weak and tired, because all the iron is taken out of their body. So they'd have that.

Margaret

After the baby's born, she's allowed to have everything from the bush. Also, from the emus, we had the oil as well to rub the body when you're in pain.

Kerry-Ann

My mum's family used to get the leaves and crush them all up and make a sticky substance. They used to just rub it on all the areas, even when the girls were pregnant too. They used to rub it around the lower back, around all of the areas where there was pain.

Dorothy

Before colonisation they would have used kangaroo skin or warm paperbark to bind the belly. They would have warmed it up and put it around because it's still like a soothing remedy that'll take the pain. You know when you've got period pain and all those pains go right down to your leg to your toes? Well, that would have helped with pain as well, so they always bound it up with kangaroo skin, dried kangaroo skin and paperbark.

They used to get big strips of paperbark and wet it and roll it up. After they'd made the fire, they'd dig all the ash and sand out and then put that in there. They'd put the sand and ash back over the top and leave it for so long until it's really warm. It's like a water bottle. My grandmother used to use a brick, or a big stone, wrap it up in a rag or something. That would be the same.

Margaret

And when we come off from having babies, we weren't allowed to wet our feet. One of the black fellas lore was you weren't allowed to put your feet in water or wet your hair.

Kerry-Ann

To keep good strong families in the Nyungar community is to try and keep our traditions and values. Breastfeeding and keeping the language strong is important: the stories, the culture and the tradition.

Dorothy

And to continue feeding the young ones traditional foods.

Ah Yi — Chinese Malaysia

I met another Teresa through her niece, Belinda, who lives in Australia. Teresa Teng has been a Chinese Malaysian confinement lady for nearly 15 years. Since I'd already interviewed Theresa, such a similar name, and because I was introduced to Teresa through her niece, I continued to call her Ah Yi (meaning *aunt*).

It was fascinating to interview someone so experienced in postpartum care in a culture where this care is the norm.

This is a really common job here in Malaysia. I have never really had to actively go in search of work. I didn't do any formal study. The only requirements of the job are to take good care of the mother. Knowledge around doing this is so common here.

Because this kind of care is so common, it is expected that all new mothers have some sort of confinement care after they give birth. We don't attend the birth itself. We just do postnatal confinement care, where we go to the new mother's home after she has given birth and then stay on to take care of her.

We work for 30 days straight, cooking for the mother, looking after the baby so that the mother can sleep and recover... basically, making sure that the baby and the mother are healthy and happy! We don't provide any medical help. If the mother or baby is sick, then we would ask for a doctor to come to the house.

It's a great way to earn money here in Malaysia and it is a job that is really important. You have to be very careful with both the baby and the mother, because they are both very vulnerable at this stage.

When you have a child, you shouldn't do work for 30 days. It's best to sleep a lot, rest and not walk around too much.

In the first week, your body is still very delicate, so you need to be gentle with it. You don't really want to be eating too much at all. But once you're into the second week, it's good to eat more and more and start building up how much you are eating.

You need to always be eating foods that are warm in constitution and in temperature during the confinement period. Make sure that all the food is well-cooked through and there is nothing raw — these are too cold for the mother.

When you have a child, your body loses a lot of its warmth, your body becomes cold and therefore needs to have its heat restored.

Additionally, the mother will have a lot of Chinese herbs and medicines to supplement her strength. These herbs can be brewed as a tea to drink, or they can be cooked into the food.

We use ginger and sesame oil in our cooking. This oil is excellent for restoring the health of the mother. It will help make the new mother stronger.

It's best to stir-fry sesame oil with ginger. It's a great base for all your cooking. You can use it in your stir-fried vegetables, you can use it to cook your meat. It's kind of sweet and delicious, and it's good for restoring the heat back into the mother's body.

Basically anything that is cold or 'windy'— that is, produces gas internally — should be avoided. So there are a lot of different foods that you can eat, but also lots of foods that you can't. You just have to be careful of the certain constitution of the foods that you are consuming.

There are always women who complain, saying, "No, I don't like this food! Why do I have to drink this medicine?" But it's really just about taking care of the woman despite all of this. It's for her own good! We have to encourage them to eat more and take more herbs by warning them of how they might get sick if they don't let us take care of them in this first month.

The women here — or Asian women in general — when we have a baby, we don't use much water. If you do use water and wash, then it's important to boil the water first and use warm water.

It's all up to the mother herself, really, but we try to not have too many showers just to minimise the chances of the mother getting cold and it's best that she doesn't wash her hair.

There is a belief that this water will go into your body and dampen your essence if you wash too much. Washing your body is generally considered to keep you in a vulnerable state rather than making you stronger and healthier. Over-washing the body is essentially a way of agitating the body's essence and distracting it from doing the healing work that it needs to do. Basically, you want to eliminate all chances of the new mother coming into contact with too many harsh elements while she is healing.

The mother needs to avoid strong winds and air conditioning too. The mother also needs to try and wear two layers of clothing if it is cold, long sleeves are preferable. Your feet also need to be very warm, so always wear socks.

It's not common for Chinese-Malaysian mothers to bind the belly. The only reason why we might bind the mother's belly would be to help her get back to her pre-baby body — to help her lose weight and get skinny — but I don't do this with the women I look after. If a mother wants this done, there is a separate professional that may come do a house call for massage and belly binding.

After one month has passed (that is, the confinement period), there is sometimes a celebration. Family and friends may give the mother red envelopes (with money for the baby and the mother) or give her other gifts, cakes etc., to celebrate the successful birth and first month of life. They might also invite all of their family and friends for a big buffet or meal to celebrate.

85

You need to integrate back into life after those 30 days really slowly too.

The women here ideally have around two months to reintegrate into daily life after they give birth. So they have a two-month holiday before they go back to work. It's generally the first month, you would be in full confinement and you would rarely leave the house. Then in the second month, you would slowly start doing a bit of work and start reintegrating. And then by the third month, you can go back to work.

The important takeaway messages from the confinement period are: you have to ensure that the new mother eats really well, she doesn't get too cold, she doesn't wash too much. Those are the main points.

For Chinese people, all women will have a confinement period. If she doesn't take care of herself after the birth, then the mother will get sick really easily. It's considered absolutely necessary. It's embedded culturally and socially. It's not really a 'trendy' thing to do... you just have to do it!

Layla — Morocco

I came across Layla B. through her work on the Nafsa Project, which aims to revive, reclaim and restore traditional Moroccan postpartum rituals and wisdom. She is a multi-passionate entrepreneur, mother, traditional postpartum trainer, writer and philanthropist. She has spent time learning from traditional midwives/healers in the north of Morocco. Here, she generously shares some of what she's learned with us.

Morocco is an interesting and amazing country. It was colonised and ruled by many different countries, hence the French, Portuguese, Spanish and Roman influences you find.

86

Even though the country is modernising very fast, luckily many traditional customs have remained and been passed down from generations. It is a diverse land with oceans, mountains, desert, beaches and snow.

I am from the north of Morocco (Tangier and Chefchaouen). Since what I share is from my own experiences, this may differ greatly to other regions.

I believe that postpartum care in Morocco is still considered essential; however, the levels vary depending on the region and the woman. Most women in Morocco will have some sort of family support at the end of their pregnancy and for about the first 40 days. Usually support is received from the mother mainly, or the mother-in-law, aunt, sister or any other female relative. The support will include caring for the new mother by allowing her to rest, cooking nourishing meals, helping with the baby if required, cleaning the home and other general tasks.

Rest is very important for the new mother in Morocco. We typically have a 40-day rest tradition where the mother should not be doing anything but resting, eating, sleeping and feeding her baby.

In more modern cities, hospital births and with women who work outside the home, it is becoming more common for them not to take up the full 40-day rest period, but it is still very common for women to rest at home and in bed and to be supported by their own mother or other female family members.

In some villages and in cases where women birth at home with a traditional qabla (midwife), they will most likely have the qabla make regular postnatal visits which include washing the mother (hamam), closing of the bones, belly binding, clearing up the house and sometimes cooking as

87

well. Of course, this differs from region to region, as some qablas in certain areas have never learned closing the bones from their elders. However, they always do the hamam and belly binding.

During the postpartum period, the new mother can go to the hamam (traditional steam bath) and her body is massaged and washed. She gets a type of massage using traditional olive soap. Some traditional midwives I've studied with also offer a 'closing' massage after the bath too.

For centuries, Moroccan women have been belly binding during the postpartum period and also during all other stages of their life. For some women, especially in villages, belly binding is an essential part of their daily life and they bind their lower belly first thing in the morning until bedtime.

The traditional midwives I have met encourage new mothers to wash their body in the shower sitting down or in the hamam, however not sitting in a bath of water. Hair can be washed, but needs to be dried and then wrapped up in a scarf to prevent any colds.

Traditionally a mother should not consume 'cold' types of food, such as cold water, cold salads and so forth. It is recommended by the traditional midwives that the new mother should consume warming and fortifying foods that allow her to recoup her strength and energy. Moroccan food generally includes a lot of warming spices such as cinnamon, ginger, turmeric and black pepper, which are great for the mother. We have a special dish that is usually not eaten on a regular basis because it is time-consuming to prepare and full of lots of herbs, spices and ingredients. This dish is called 'rfissa', normally served best with organic free-range chicken cooked in a sauce of onions, lentils, herbs, garlic and a famous spice mix called 'ras al hanoot', which includes about 30 different warming spices blended together. The chicken is served on top of a bed of homemade 'ftayar' (a type of bread, but made very thinly and then chopped into pieces). Boiled eggs are scattered around and the chicken soup is served alongside it.

The most 'famous' postpartum herb for mothers in Morocco is lemon balm. The mother is advised to sit on it in the hamam or use it for steaming. We also use a lot of lavender, rosemary, myrtle, sage and mint. We have the famous Moroccan tea with mint, which is consumed throughout the day in most households. During the postpartum, other herbs such as lemon verbena, thyme, wormwood and sage can be added in. A lot of amazing olive oil is produced in Morocco, so this is definitely the go-to oil. It is used in cooking, for the 'closing' massage, during birth and for anything else.

The postpartum mother is very much advised to keep warm in order to heal and recover properly, and not to catch any 'colds', which could affect her in later life.

During home births, the mother is surrounded by blankets at all times, after birth as well, and she is advised not to eat or drink anything cold, not to shower in cold water, to wear long clothes and cover her hair even after the first 40 days is over.

I remember when the traditional midwife visited me after the birth of my last baby, I was way over 40 days and wearing trousers and a t-shirt. The midwife was shocked and told me that I had to cover my elbows and knees at all times since the cold would go through there. It was the middle of summer and she was wearing leggings, warm socks on top, covered hair, multiple layers and her belly was bound!

Traditionally, the placenta is buried in the ground or in a plant, never thrown in the bin and never eaten.

When people knew their neighbours and lived in smaller villages, the women would take turns to cook meals and bring them round to the new mother, and help her out at home if needed.

In Morocco, we have the 'aqiqa', also known as the seventh day, which stems from an Islamic celebration to welcome the new baby and mother. Family, friends and neighbours are usually invited to eat together and celebrate. The baby is normally named and guests bring gifts, sometimes for the baby only or for the mother too.

The 'aqiqa' is not specifically to initiate the new mother. However, traditionally, the new mother was treated like a bride; because brides in Morocco go through months of planning, preparation and pampering. The new mother would be served for at least 40 days. She would be taken to the hamam with a crew of other women. Candles, sweets, food and lots of singing would take place on the journey to the hamam and inside. She would then be taken home and have henna applied on her hands and feet. Normally there would be a small party at home and they would eat 'rfissa' together. The new mother would also get closing of her bones, shown how to belly-bind, washed, pampered and nourished for the whole of the 40 days.

That is their celebration and initiation to motherhood, which is delightful!

Naomie - Giriama tribe in Kenya

Naomie Karemi is a doula from Kenya currently living in the Netherlands. I met Naomie online and was delighted when she agreed to share some traditional postpartum practices from her Giriama people.

We [the Giriama people] *don't have doulas exactly, but old midwives called wa-kunga. Wa is plural in Swahili. A traditional midwife is called mkunga. My own grandmother was a mkunga and she helped deliver quite a lot of my cousins. They live in an area within communities where hospitals are far away and so birth skills are passed from generation to generation. In the villages, they do postpartum care as well. It is tradition.*

Where I'm from - the Giriama tribe - it's traditional that women all give birth under the same sacred tree. The child is normally anointed. The mum would sometimes go back and hang a piece of cloth on the tree that looks like a flag in the name of their child to show appreciation to the ancestors who guided the birth and protected the child's journey, so it's beautifully decorated.

There is belief that how the placenta is handled will determine the fertility for the mother in the future. The placenta leaves the hut according to the sex of the baby born. It leaves the birthing hut from the right for a baby boy, and the left for a baby girl. The placenta is planted with a tree within the community. The family choose a spot within their communal ground where they want to plant it. It's a celebration. We are giving back to mother earth. The community would gather together for it. There are songs and drumbeats. Wine is poured on the ground as an offering for the ancestors that have gone before us, and then the placenta is buried. The mother would bless and release the placenta and the father would bury it.

In Kenya, the postpartum period starts when the woman is six months pregnant. That's when the women actually gather together to prepare the mother-to-be for the birth. The woman would move back to her mother's or in-laws' where she would get continuous support, because the people believe highly in that support.

Before a woman gets married, we have kitchen parties. When a daughter gets her first period, her godmother buys her first pads and initiates the one to one moment to explain what this new phase means, personal hygiene etc. These are traditions that have been passed down. It's the same during postpartum with women who have the experience coming together to pass on the knowledge and say, "You're going to be okay because there is a whole herd of us behind you."

They come offering gifts of the feminine world. We have a wrap called a kanga that you see a lot of African women wrap between the waist and the shoulders. A kanga is used for the birth, and you use it again for carrying the baby afterwards. It's like a tool that every woman in the traditional communities has in their bag. In case you have that period you didn't expect, you have a kanga to cover you. It's like the essential cloth that you can have as a woman. With the kanga, we normally have a sort of closing ceremony and we also use it for belly binding.

My mum still had the kanga from when I was born and she brought it to me when I had my first daughter. My mum came for both my births in Amsterdam to do the 40-day celebration. I was in bed at home and she just did everything. She came for three months both times. I had the most amazing postpartum period!

I have supported many families now in Holland. You get eight days of the Kraamzorg [postnatal care service], *but they are more serious about the number of diapers that the baby has peed in and checking the mum's incision, rather than the real personalised care. Plus, it's only eight days. The fathers go back to work quickly and it's not long enough, so mothers feel left out and alone. It's quite a shock, as a new mum you have to stagger about and think what to feed yourself for this child who is clinging onto you for breast milk.*

I met a woman once in the pharmacy when my daughter peeped through the pram and said, "Oh Mama, look, there's a cute little baby inside." I looked over, greeted the mother, and said, "How are you?" And she broke down crying. It's tough.

In Kenya at the moment you become a mother, you are a queen. There are facial masks, head massages, joint massages, henna is drawn on the legs or the hands, but there is also a rub that is done. We call it liwa and it's made from sandalwood and turmeric that is rubbed with water and a bit of oil, then smeared on you. Then you are wrapped up using Kangas or Kikoi. Meanwhile the baby is looked after, from hand to hand amongst the helpers around you

For 40 days, the mother is in exclusion and the only people who are allowed to come and visit her are the immediate family: the husband, the grandparents, and such like. Not neighbours and friends. Everybody else respects that.

During the 40 days, she's not really restricted to staying in bed, but she is not allowed to do anything heavy that will hinder her recovery. Sex is not allowed during this recovery period. She's not expected to do any chores, food is cooked for her, she's looked after and the baby's being looked after too.

The basic ugali flour is what we give all birthing mothers because it helps produce enough milk. It's the cake that we make from maize meal. It's basic and has no flavour. It's

93

heavy enough to keep you going for hours on end but not so heavy that it's draining. We don't touch stuff like beef because that's too heavy.

The main meal will be ugali, with a stew with free-range chicken and some vegetables. In a lot of the homesteads, you'll find quite a lot of greenery around, and they love to eat from their own ground, often spinach, kale, and okra. Mums will be given stuff like that to help with bowel movements. Mums also eat lentils that have normally been soaked the night before so they're not gassy when eaten. Red kidney beans are not given because gas is inevitable! We use a lot of mung beans and coconut milk too.

We make bread like pancakes called chapati from meal that is also made nearby. Most village people harvest their own grains and they take them to a mill where it's turned to meal powder. They begin to prepare the grains when the mother is still pregnant.

So that the mother stays the same body temperature, she would be wiped down, not washed fully in the bathroom. We normally wrap the legs a lot so that she's not exposed to cold. And if she's grown up in the city, they would normally say, "Make sure you put your socks on" because cold travels from the feet up. You are wrapped from head to toes because it is believed that when you birth, women open up completely during birth including their heads which is the Chakra. Coconut oil is normally mixed with water before massaged in the scalp because water penetrates the skin better. To wade off any headaches and to relax your mind.

We have the 40-day ceremony after birth and after death. It's the same sacred passage. For some they call the 40+4 and some do 40+10 days. A refresher kitchen party is organised to refresh the new mother on her new role as a mother and wife. Whatever she was taught for her marriage is topped up for life with a child, like how she is not allowed to soak dirty nappies till they stink the house down.

Kenyan communities have openness with the women and the 40-day celebration is where the honesty comes in. For a bride, we talk about Kama Sutra. And for a mother, we talk about fanny farts! We've all been there! It's not going to be easy, but these are things that she needs to make sure that she's doing, because they are for her benefit and for her marriage.

The closing ceremony is initiated with the mum and the baby. When I had my daughter, that was the day she was named, the day I was reminded I was out of absolute danger, the day I was encouraged to let my tears flow, my worries go, and give thanks to your womb for granting you the honour of carrying a pregnancy to fruition till birth, my daughter's hair was shaved off, and then the blessing started from the door. Everything is blessed on the doorstep. A bride is also blessed at the entrance; coffins are placed next to the door. Everything. I remember when my son was born with health issues on my blessing day my mother reminding me to still honour and give thanks that I had given birth

For the 40-day ceremony, the baby's right ear is normally held by the grandparent and wisdom is spoken to them. The mum is blessed by being drenched from head to toe. It's the first proper wash and she's allowed to wash her hair too, she's allowed to have water penetrate all the holes in her body. That's the moment that she steps out in the community. From that start, she has to be strong enough to continue.

Reviving Your Family Legacy

Sometimes it's easier to look outside of our own culture for wisdom and it might feel as though these traditions are exotic but in my experience, beautiful postpartum traditions exist in every culture! It's just a matter of when and how much they have been eroded by colonisation, globalisation and the patriarchy.

If you can, I invite you to ask your mother or your grandmothers or any other non-related elders from your own cultural background to share their postpartum stories and traditions with you.

Who knows what secret women's business and pearls of wisdom you will uncover, and what legacy you can revive.

Traditions

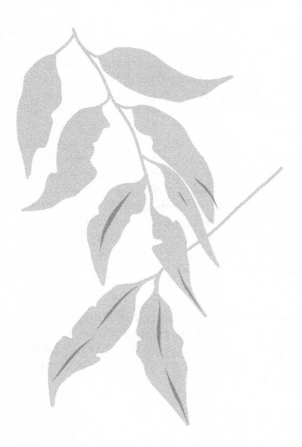

40 Days For 40 Years

In many cultures, there is a distinct and significant time after birth, where the mother is considered to have unique needs and require a special kind of care. We know there are good reasons for this; the early weeks and months are a time of great change, when patterns are established that may affect a mother and her family for many years to come.

Physically, it takes roughly six to eight weeks for your breast milk supply to establish and become regulated. While it took 40 weeks for your uterus to expand with your growing baby, it takes only 40 days to contract down to its original size and for the bleeding to stop after birth. Emotionally, it is also a time of high brain plasticity and increased oxytocin.

Special care during this time is observed traditionally in hundreds of cultures all over the world. In England in Victorian times, women expected what they called *confinement* after giving birth, in fact some hospitals today still refer to EDC — estimated date of confinement! In China, it's known as *doing the month or sitting the month*. In Spanish speaking countries, the specific time after birth is known as *la cuarentena*, meaning 'the forty'. In Brazil, I've heard of *double care*, meaning care for the mother as well as the baby.

In many cultures, there are layers and stages: a time spent in bed, a time spent indoors, a time when visitors are restricted, and eventually a time when daily responsibilities officially resume and a mother is welcomed into her new role by her community.

Ysha Oakes first introduced me to the concept of '40 days for 40 years'. It represents the belief that the right care and support during this stage of your life can set you up for health and love for many years to come. Those first 40 days after childbirth are a unique invitation for deep healing, growth and initiation.

Likewise, neglect during this time can lead to long-term mental, physical and emotional health problems, sometimes even years after your babies have grown up.

What if I Missed my 40 Days?

If you are pregnant, this is a perfect time to be reading this book and planning for your peaceful and joyful postpartum. I'll show you exactly how to do this.

But if you have already had your baby, it's likely your 40 days were not what you hoped or expected. Our culture is so suspicious and afraid of childbirth that during pregnancy we are typically fixated on this one aspect. As a result, we spend little time preparing pregnant women for the weeks and months afterwards.

In case you missed your 40 days, don't panic. While postpartum offers a rare biological opportunity, remember how your brain can change in response to your environment too? If you are feeling overwhelmed and exhausted, it's never too late to change your environment, and to rewire your brain for peace and joy.

I invite you to do some baby-brain-boosting, some village-building and receive postpartum care right now, no matter how old your baby is. Enriching your environment will enrich your brain.

What if I Don't Want to Stay Home for 40 Days?

Some strong and independent women rally against the idea of confinement and may find all the rules and restrictions suffocating and patronising. In cultures where these traditions are still practised, some Newborn Mothers reject them as superstitious and old-fashioned. For extroverted women, there may be feelings of loneliness if they are forced to stay home without visitors for defined periods of time.

At times, these postpartum traditions have been corrupted by the patriarchy as a way of infantilising or controlling women, but originally they were designed to support new mothers. This is why I'm not a big fan of rules and regulations. I'm sure there are enough people telling you what you should and shouldn't be doing right now.

Instead, understand the intention and meaning of these care practices, and how to make them relevant and appealing to you. I aim to encourage you to embrace the idea that love conquers all, and to create a specific period of peace and joy, whatever that looks like for you.

When creating your postpartum plan or making decisions ask yourself *how does this feel for me?*

Barriers to Peace and Joy During Your 40 Days

Sometimes you create the best postpartum plans, only to find the reality utterly different. Even when pregnant women are aware of the value of planning for postpartum, I've noticed there are three major barriers stopping them from getting the care they want after having a baby.

The first and most common barrier is inside your head. Even when you know that postpartum is an important time, there is gap between intellectual knowledge and deep understanding. You may still have subconscious stories about work that make you feel guilty and lazy when you rest. Or perhaps you are trying to DIY because the thought of asking for help is unbearable! The stillness and silence of 40 days' rest is a perfect opportunity for you to re-examine your belief systems, and decide if they will serve you and your family well in the future.

Then there is the difficulty of changing gears. As Kerstin Uvnäs Moberg pointed out, our culture values challenge, competition and performance, making it hard to adjust your habits and thinking to a slower pace of life. Motherhood may feel boring by comparison, and you may crave more novelty and adventure. Depending on your personality and temperament, you might be able to surrender into it as a brief stage, knowing it will pass. Or maybe you could find a way to socialise with visitors in your own gregarious and fun way, whilst still resting at home in your pyjamas and refraining from housework. Or perhaps you may find you can push through the boredom to find a more peaceful and tranquil way of life in the longer term.

And finally, of course, there are social, financial and cultural barriers. Maybe you don't have adequate maternity leave, or enough support from friends and family. Maybe people think you are crazy for doing your 40 days differently. Wisdom is knowing what you can change. While there may be certain aspects of your situation that you have to accept, there is always something you can change. Focus on that. Give yourself the best chance of postpartum peace and joy by working on your mindset, and surrounding yourself with a community of like-minded mothers.

Rest

With so little support and understanding of postpartum, it's common for Newborn Mothers to just get on with normal daily life after having a baby. We are encouraged to act as though nothing has really changed, when on the inside, everything feels completely different.

In many parts of the world, rest is literally mandated for Newborn Mothers! In some cultures, mothers are told to lie in bed for days or even weeks, and absolutely not allowed to exercise. During this time, she is seen as vulnerable and sensitive, just like her new baby. She is often cosseted and coddled; sometimes fed with a spoon like a baby and sometimes not allowed to leave her bedroom, even to go to the toilet.

Unsurprisingly, problems arise when traditions are forced upon a mother against her will. Some mothers rebel against these prohibitions. Some more introverted mothers relish the idea of hibernating with their baby for an extended period of time. Other more extroverted mothers prefer to go for short walks in nature and meet friends at cafes.

The essence of the idea is to nourish and nurture the mother, so she can nourish and nurture her baby. You need to do what nourishes and nurtures you.

And that, naturally, looks different for everyone.

Your Only Two Jobs Are Falling in Love and Learning to Breastfeed

In order to support deep and extended rest, around the world Newborn Mothers are protected from household work like cooking and cleaning, paid work, and religious duties such fasting or attending church.

You would be expected to rest and heal. Your only two jobs would be learning to breastfeed and falling in love. That may sound like a fantasy to you, but it is surprisingly common around the world.

And if there's anything else that is taking your time and energy away from your two jobs — falling in love and learning to breastfeed — ideally your community would step in and take care of it for you. Since we've lost that framework, you're going to need to be courageous and ask for help yourself.

It Takes Time to Fall in Love

Some mothers experience love-at-first-sight when they meet their babies. But I've worked with other women in the early days after giving birth who feel terrible guilt and shame because they have not experienced an ecstatic moment of falling in love with their baby.

In the movies, it looks so instant and absolute.

In reality, for some women, it feels more like an arranged marriage.

Who is this person!?

103

There seems to be this mythology that bonding is a blink-and-you'll-miss-it moment, a fragile and time-sensitive process with certain ritualised actions a mother must take or else bonding will not occur. But bonding is simply falling in love; and building a relationship with any human being can take time.

We create a secure attachment with our children by being present and responsive to their needs, not necessarily by having a natural birth or breastfeeding or co-sleeping or babywearing. It is not so much what you do, but how you do it. Your baby will be securely attached when you parent with loving and mindful presence, regardless of your situation or parenting choices.

Enjoy your baby, spend time with your baby, listen to your baby.

Before you know it, your heart will be so full of love it may feel like it's going to burst.

And here is the biggest challenge, in order to find the time it takes to bond with your baby, you'll need to let go of the superwoman myth and ask for help with other jobs in your life.

It Takes a Village to Breastfeed

Humans have been successfully breastfeeding for thousands of years, but today only one in three mothers meets her own breastfeeding goals.[1]

Women want to breastfeed, but something is going terribly wrong. And when it's such a widespread problem, we need to stop blaming individual mothers and start looking at the bigger picture.

When a mother struggles to breastfeed, our culture's typical response is masculine: to look for problems to fix and solve, to give advice and pass judgement. Women are usually given information, charts, diagrams and routines. Mothers are told to weigh babies and bottles of milk and introduce breast pumps and formula.

Sometimes these strategies might be helpful, but I don't think it should be our first port of call. My suggestion is radically different.

Generally, when a mother is struggling to breastfeed, the first place I look is to her support networks. Who is cooking and cleaning for you? Are you getting enough rest and nutrition? Do you have other people caring for your older children? Are the people around you sabotaging breastfeeding because they have little experience of breastfeeding themselves?

Breastfeeding is literally a full-time job! In those early weeks, a baby can feed every hour or two around the clock, often for 30 to 40 minutes at a time. Do the maths. That's easily eight or nine hours a day with a baby attached to your breast!

Often when a mother expresses her breastfeeding challenges, what she is really feeling is *I had no idea it would be this intense; I must be doing something wrong; I'm a failure.*

You are not a failure. Breastfeeding is natural, but it is also a learned skill and a difficult one at that. We need to stop thinking of breastfeeding as a photo on Instagram and start seeing it as a marathon. When someone is running a marathon and they say it's hard and they're tired, what do we do? We cheer them on. *You can do it! You're halfway there! One foot in front of the other! You're doing great!*

105

Breastfeeding is a big job. It's messy and unpredictable and challenging and rewarding and wonderful.

If you want to breastfeed, you'll turn the odds in your favour by building your village. In order to have plenty of time to breastfeed, you'll need practical and emotional support, which brings me to the topic of exactly who can provide you with that support.

The Origins of Doulas

Anthropologist Dana Raphael was looking for an answer to why breastfeeding was so difficult for women in our culture after being disappointed by her own personal experience. She explored nearly 200 different cultures and found similar postpartum care patterns occurring universally. What she found is profound:

"I had discovered that there was a physiological process (breastfeeding) that needed to have something in place in the culture or else the lactation function would not work. I don't know of any other biological process that needs the culture to supply support... If you don't have that support, usually you cannot feed your baby."[2]

Dana Raphael went on to coin the word 'doula' — in its modern sense — to mean breastfeeding support person. She says that she was talking about her discovery when she was overheard by an elderly Greek woman who said, "Oh yes, that's a doula."

In fact, the Greek origins of the word *doula* are dubious, but many cultures have a specific name for the role of a doula: *dai* in India, *handywoman* in England, *pui yuet* in China. Yet the name *doula* persisted in English langauge.

Over time, our industrialised hospital system has meant that doulas have stepped into the birthing room to offer emotional and practical support there. The word is now synonymous with a birth support person.

It still stands that support massively improves your chances of being able to breastfeed as well. Traditionally, this support may have come from a friend or family member. The problem we face in our culture is that, even though our friends and family want to help, they don't actually know how. Since they're not really familiar with a Newborn Mother's needs and postpartum traditions, they can actually do more harm than good.

And that's why postpartum doulas are gaining popularity.

What Exactly Does a Postpartum Doula do?

Postpartum doulas, like me, are non-medical professionals designed to fill the postpartum-shaped gap in maternal care. We provide emotional and physical support during the life-changing transition to motherhood and help women step into their new roles with confidence and satisfaction.

Of course, every doula is different, and every mother has different needs and expectations, but here are some general ways a postpartum doula might work with you.

Your postpartum doula will support you and your family in bonding with your baby by encouraging you to spend time together. We facilitate the process of gaining a deeper understanding of your baby's personality and temperament and developing confidence in your unique parenting style.

Postpartum doulas typically provide companionship and emotional support by actively listening, providing a shoulder

107

to cry on or having a cup of tea and a laugh together. You can literally ask us anything! There are no questions too big, too small or too embarrassing for a postpartum doula.

In order to empower you and your partner in your choices, your postpartum doula may provide evidence-based information regarding basic baby care and normal breastfeeding. A good postpartum doula will always make referrals where appropriate.

Having a baby is a big transition for everyone and we also provide support for partners, siblings and extended family during the adjustment period. We understand the dynamics of all relationships will be affected and support positive communication.

Your postpartum doula will help you build your village by connecting you with classes, groups and other professionals. Many families need support managing visitors, extended family, friends and neighbours, including setting boundaries.

Your postpartum doula will encourage self-care and asking for help, and provide physical and practical support including light cleaning and cooking nutritious meals for the whole family.

Every doula is different, and most will adjust each visit to suit your specific needs on that day. And many postpartum doulas have other specialised skills too, like massage or herbs or traditional cultural care, so you are sure to find one who suits you.

Nourishing Comfort Food

When I was writing my recipe book *Nourishing Newborn Mothers*, a few people told me they wanted recipes for foods they could cook and eat one-handed, but that wasn't what I had in mind.

Postpartum food around the world is designed to be cooked for you, not by you. Food cooked fresh by people who love you has the ability to heal you on a much deeper and more subtle level than food that you've struggled to cook and eat alone with one hand whilst breastfeeding, wrangling your toddler and talking on the phone.

All over the world, women are given special food after the baby is born. This food varies in the details according to the customs and staple foods of each culture, but there are a few universal patterns I have noticed.

Food Taboos

Food taboos and dietary restrictions are common, and ideas about what mothers should and shouldn't eat vary a lot, and often contradict each other. They vary from country to country, and village to village, and they change over time.

Many of these dietary restrictions are easy to dismiss as superstitious, like "eating eggs will make your baby smelly" or "eating snails will make your baby lazy". But don't assume that mothers in more affluent and educated areas are immune to advice about the perils of eating while breastfeeding. I've met many stressed-out Australian mothers with lists of foods they can't eat as long as their arm and they feel terrified that anything they put in their mouth will cause their baby gas or keep them awake or make them cry...

So why do we have all these rules?

It's possible that these postpartum rituals have evolved to bring the extended family together to rally around the new mother and her baby during this important time. It's simply a way for potential alloparents to show you that they care about your baby. Indeed, postpartum diets are often so strict that a Newborn Mother couldn't possibly be expected to remember all the rules and prepare her own food! Complex food taboos create a system of nurturing, community and support around the new family.

However, in some less developed parts of the world, such strict food restrictions can actually do harm since the mothers are not getting their nutritional needs met. While there is less danger of this happening in developed countries, no matter what you eat, your body is quite determined to make high quality milk for your baby. If your diet is lacking in energy and nutrition, your milk will be prioritised and made from your body's stores. So though your baby will be able to survive your deprivation diet just fine, you are more likely to suffer depletion in the long run.

You've possibly already received a bewildering array of suggestions on foods to avoid, but in fact there is no food that all breastfeeding mothers should avoid. When balancing up the risks and benefits of eliminating certain foods from your diet, here are a few things to consider.

Is your diet reducing your ability to socialise, eat out or have friends and family cook for you? Is your diet causing you anxiety and stress? Is your diet preventing you from eating a balanced range of healthy foods? Is your diet so difficult to maintain that you are feeling discouraged from breastfeeding?

Now, certain babies *are* sensitive to particular foods, but every baby is unique, and I suggest you listen to your baby and no one else.

But before we throw the baby out with the bathwater...

What to Eat

I love food so much I've devoted an entire book to recipes that can heal your mind, body and soul after childbirth. And I prefer to focus on the positive: what to eat rather than what not to eat.

Here are some universal, nourishing themes I've found when examining postpartum diets from a variety of cultures.

Many traditional medicine systems are generally based on the elements — earth, fire, water and wind — and this usually gives new mothers guidance on what to eat. For example, when you are pregnant, you generally feel hot, heavy and wet, but after your baby is born, you more likely feel cold, dry and light. You would be encouraged to eat foods that are opposite to the elements in your body, for balance.

This is the kind of language often used to explain postpartum foods, but in case you aren't familiar with traditional medicine, let me translate for you.

As a Newborn Mother, you need a lot of energy to breastfeed, recover from pregnancy and birth, and cope with sleep deprivation. Many postpartum foods are designed to build blood, increase milk supply, and also to strengthen and heal the body after pregnancy and childbirth.

Warm, nourishing, comfort foods are a worldwide theme. Soups, stews and puddings are common features on

111

international postpartum menus, which often resemble what you would feed babies or invalids. In general, foods are rich, sweet and easy to digest.

Chicken soup, rice pudding, porridge, herbal tea and hot chocolate are all examples of soothing, comforting foods that are popular around the world. As postpartum is already a time of great change, it's not a good time to be making drastic changes to your diet.

Instead, you need familiarity, so add your personal favourite 'soup for the soul' type recipes to your postpartum plan.

Staying Warm

For similar reasons, it's common for cultures around the world to put a lot of effort into warming up Newborn Mothers.

There are many different ways of doing this, but most cultures have some way of applying warmth to the mother's body. Examples include daily massages with warm oil or hot stones, saunas, smoking ceremonies and simply keeping mothers protected from draughts and wind.

It may be possible that physical warmth is thought to increase emotional warmth, that cosiness in our environment makes us feel more generous, sensitive and caring.

One of my favourite words for postpartum is the Danish word *hygge*. Pronounced *hoo-guh*, it means a 'quality of cosiness and comfortable conviviality that engenders a feeling of contentment or wellbeing'[3]. Hygge also implies a warm and welcoming social atmosphere, which means no conflict or judgment, and no discussing politics or economics. Hygge means spending time with loved ones and creating a refuge or safe haven.

Ways to add more warmth to your postpartum plan include: candles, pots of tea, cooked foods, snuggly blankets and comfy socks.

No Washing

In many cultures, women are forbidden from bathing or washing their hair for certain periods after giving birth. This is definitely one of the less popular postpartum traditions! There are a few possible reasons why this might have been a helpful idea for Newborn Mothers once-upon-a-time, but lucky for you it may not be relevant anymore.

The first is hygiene. Throughout much of human history access to clean water was limited. After childbirth is a vulnerable time for a mother. Your immunity may be lower than usual and you may have cracked nipples, and open cuts and tears from the birth. Showering in dirty water is potentially dangerous.

The second reason is that in the past the water available would often have been cold. It's only relatively recently that humans have had hot water on demand, and well-heated homes! And since getting cold was discouraged, showering and bathing was discouraged too.

The third reason is to promote breastfeeding. Newborn babies have a good sense of smell, and use it to recognise you and initiate breastfeeding.[4] When your baby does the breast-crawl to find your milk, he literally uses smell to guide himself to your nipple. Perhaps there's a reason that your armpits are so close to your breasts!

If you have access to clean and hot water, obviously feel free to wash as often as you like, but consider skipping smelly soaps and perfumes if you plan to breastfeed. Your baby loves your unique scent.

Massage

It's likely you know that touch, skin-on-skin and massage are excellent for newborn babies, but it's unlikely anyone mentioned they are great for Newborn Mothers too.

In many traditional cultures, massage was a part of standard postpartum care. There are many different kinds including breast massage, uterus massage and 'closing of the bones'. Massages often include the application of herbal pastes, warm compresses or hot stones.

It's fairly easy to imagine why postpartum massage is popular around the world. It supports some of the other traditions, like warming the body and encouraging deep rest. It also improves metabolism and circulation during a time without exercise. Massage also increases oxytocin.

And many traditional postpartum massages end with binding the mother's beautiful belly...

Belly binding

No matter how many gimmicky websites on the internet tell you so, there's absolutely no evidence that belly binding will help you lose weight. However, it's a powerful postpartum practice nonetheless and it's being embraced by more and more mothers today.

In Malaysia, it's called *beng kung*, and in Mexico they use *rebozo*. Many different cultures bind new mothers' bellies, and while it may sound a bit like a torturous corset, this is not the intention at all!

Belly binding can support your posture while your core muscles and pelvic floor are still recovering and not yet

114

strong. It aids the application of herbs and oils, which are often applied after massage, then the belly binding holds it all in place, so they can slowly be absorbed.

Often right after giving birth, particularly if you've had more babies, your skin and muscles can feel overstretched and loose and your organs feel like they are swishing around inside a washing machine! Belly binding supports the internal organs during those early weeks.

But most of all, it *feels* really good.

Deep pressure can feel grounding and supportive and like an all-day hug! Sometimes it can make you feel more at home inside a body that may otherwise feel quite foreign.

If you want to try out belly binding make sure the binding is firm and even, and doesn't dig in to your sensitive and soft belly. The binding should go from your ribs to your hips so your bones provide a frame for even pressure to be distributed across your entire abdomen.

However, I have worked with some mothers who don't enjoy the feeling of belly binding, so as always, be guided by your body and do what brings you peace and joy.

Initiation

Do you feel special when you're pregnant? I certainly did. People would give me their seat on the train, offer to carry my heavy bags and hold the door open for me.

I remember when I was pregnant the man at the post office carried my parcel out to my car for me, but when I turned up at the same post office a few months later with my newborn and my toddler, I had to carry my own parcel!

It was as though my body was sacred and respected only while my baby was inside me, but as soon as the baby was born that attention remained on the baby and I was relegated to backstage.

I realised that even our gifts, including toys and clothes, and celebrations like baby showers and christenings are all centred around the baby, not the mother.

But becoming a mother is a huge life transition, and some cultures acknowledge this rite of passage with gifts and celebrations to welcome you into your new role. In some parts of the world, there are one-month celebrations, 100-day ceremonies, coming-out-of-the-house parties, and rituals like head-shaving and henna.

My favourite example of initiation of a mother comes from Uganda.

"Three months after the birth of her child, the Chagga woman's head is shaved and crowned with a bead tiara, she is robed in an ancient skin garment worked with beads, a staff such as the elders carry is put in her hand, and she emerges from her hut for the first public appearance with her baby. Proceeding slowly towards the market, they are greeted with songs such as are sung to warriors returning from battle."[5]

You don't need to shave your head or sing warrior songs. Maybe henna isn't part of your culture. All of these are simply symbols.

You are probably going through the biggest personal transformation of your entire life. A little acknowledgement of this can be a great source of satisfaction and pride. However you choose to celebrate this, ideally you would feel strong, respected, capable and confident.

Six weeks is traditionally when your confinement ends. It's time to rejoin the world.

Expanding the Postpartum Window

It's quite possible, particularly if you've had a rough time for any reason, that six weeks is not long enough. It's also likely you have periods of restlessness when you've wanted to get back into life more quickly. You may feel great while resting at home, but then overdo it by going to a busy event or taking on too many responsibilities. Don't think of these as setbacks or failures; often there's some back and forth while you find your balance. Just listen to your body and adjust accordingly.

Take it slowly. Even if you think you should be able to do more, start with short visits to your local park in good weather. Take a friend or family member with you to help you with figuring out how to unfold the pram and deal with inevitable poo explosions. You may find large crowds and department stores overwhelming, and there is a good reason for this. You are a Newborn Mother, as sensitive and vulnerable as your baby; if you find it overwhelming imagine how your baby feels! You are your baby's barometer.

You may need to rest at home for longer in case you had a difficult birth or inadequate support or still haven't gotten the hang of breastfeeding. You may need to return to nourishing, comfort foods during hectic periods for years after having your baby. Housework and sleep deprivation will only increase with more children, so you'll need to ask for help in the long term.

In fact, it's essential that we start to expand the idea of postpartum, and recognise that women are vulnerable for many years after childbirth, and we need long-term support in our roles as mothers.

Animal studies show persistent changes in mothers' brains and behaviours that last beyond weaning and even into old age! Small human studies have found that changes in grey matter endure for at least two years postpartum, and the study didn't measure beyond that.[6]

A recent longitudinal study of over 1,500 women found that maternal depression is more common four years after your baby is born than at any time during the first year of your baby's life![7]

Postpartum simply means *after birth*. You will always be postpartum. You will always be a mother, and as a mother, you will always need your village and the courage to ask for help.

Reality Check

As an outsider, it's easy to see traditional postpartum care with rose-coloured glasses. From a distance, we could romanticise faraway places and lament times gone by. In fact, many people have hypothesised that traditional postpartum care is protective against postpartum depression.

If only it were that simple!

Sadly in many parts of the world traditional postpartum care has been eroded by colonisation, globalisation and the patriarchy. In reality, a global literature review by the World Health Organisation found that depression during pregnancy or after childbirth affects two to three times more women in developing countries than in industrialised countries. Major factors contributing to maternal mental health are strikingly similar around the world — regardless of postpartum care — and include relationship quality, physical health, poverty, access to education, family-friendly employment, obstetric experience, personal safety and reproductive autonomy.[8]

It is vital that we work together to improve women's rights everywhere, in a holistic way.

But on a more individual level, while postpartum care may sometimes be protective, it seems that ritualised care that "imposes control and restricts the woman's autonomy might actually be harmful".[8]

Ultimately, it comes down to not only support, but also self-determination.

Even the most beautiful and nourishing practices can become strict rules, and this kind of rigidity defeats the original nurturing intention of the practices. For example, you may be encouraged to eat a particular food, even if you dislike it, or you feel you are not supposed to wash your hair, even when you really want to.

For ultimate postpartum peace and joy, you need the freedom to choose.

Instead of getting stuck on details or research or routines or methods, tune into your body and figure out what feels good for you, because if it feels good, it's probably increasing your oxytocin.

Take what works, and leave what doesn't.

The criteria that I want you to analyse all your postpartum decisions against is simply: does it bring you peace and joy?

Bringing it all together

Have you noticed? I've been dropping a few hints along the way…

Nourishing comfort food came up in this book in both my discussion of baby brain and of traditional care. Massage and belly binding feature in ritual postpartum care, and loving touch also increases oxytocin. Warmth is both related to oxytocin release and considered critical for Newborn Mothers in traditional cultures around the world.

Resting, cosiness, yummy food and good friends... the ancient wisdom is backed up by the latest brain science! While traditional medicine might use concepts like 'fire' and 'water' and 'space', perhaps we are still talking about the exact same ideas.

Our ancestors — without brain scans or peer-reviewed studies or doctorates — understood the profound changes you are going through when you become a mother. They figured out ways of supporting Newborn Mothers through this process.

And now you know too.

So what are you going to do about it?

Renaissance

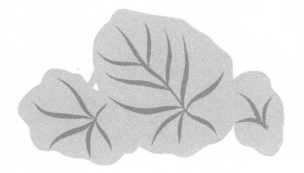

Join the Renaissance

It's happening right now, all over the world. In the decade I've been doing postpartum work, I've seen the rise and rise of mothers everywhere. The internet has given us a voice and an audience that we've never had access to before, and our stories are finally being shared and heard in a much bigger way.

Newborn Mothers everywhere are realising that we are not alone. In the past, mothers were expected to grit their teeth and bear the immense workload without emotional or practical support. If they dared ask for help, they may have been labelled hysterical, or given 'Mother's Little Helper', been institutionalised, or occasionally even had their children removed.

While some of these attitudes still persist, the landscape is changing fast. But the only way we can change it is together.

This is your invitation to join the renaissance, a revolution in your heart and your home. As you expand your life in peace and joy, you are inviting other mothers to join you in peace and joy too.

Together we can create a new blueprint for motherhood.

Here's how.

The Six Pillars of Postpartum Peace and Joy

I know you are tired. I know you don't have much time. I know you're probably still finding your way around your new brain. So I'm going to make this really simple for you.

I've distilled this new postpartum paradigm into six pillars, designed to lift you up, and bring other mothers up with you. These pillars are the essence of what you've learned so far, refined in a more simple, actionable and practical way.

This is your Newborn Mothers manifesto.

Are you ready?

1. Make a Plan

A postpartum plan is usually where most pregnant women start, and it's a great start. But the problem with planning for postpartum before you actually have a baby is that you don't know what you don't know.

It's easy to write a list of equipment you might need like a cot and a pram and car seat. You could also jot down some ideas for traditional postpartum care like belly binding and baby massage. You might choose to rest at home for a few weeks and have regular massages. I'd also encourage you to ask your elders to share their postpartum wisdom, and invite your friends to fill your freezer with nourishing comfort food.

These are all excellent ideas.

But you don't yet know who you are going to be as a mother. You haven't met your baby yet. You don't know how the birth will turn out.

123

Be flexible and curious in your methods whilst focussed on your intention of peace and joy. Be prepared to change the plan if things don't turn out the way you'd imagined. Adjust, adapt, accept. Don't get stuck in an information frenzy, there's more to postpartum then planning.

Make a plan, but don't stick to it.

2. Build Your Village

As a new mother, it's possible that you've never been less alone, and never been more lonely. It is one of the many paradoxes of motherhood. Motherhood is messy and challenging, but when you surround yourself with the right people, it can also be deeply rewarding and satisfying.

That said, many women are surprised to find their mothers' group is judgmental and competitive, when what you are really looking for is inspiration and support.

The right people will lift you up, not drag you down.

Seek out that safe space where your differences are not a source of defensiveness or insecurity, but are celebrated as innovation and creativity as each individual mother finds solutions that work for her unique family.

When you find this encouragement and understanding, you will be able to make positive changes in your life so much more quickly, and your profound growth will inspire and motivate other mothers too.

Find your village, and spend lots of time there.

3. Make Mistakes

There is a reason babies don't come with a manual! Every baby is different, and every mother is different, and every family is different.

That's why you won't find what you need in an information frenzy. In fact, when there's too much outside noise, it can be hard to connect with your baby. There is only one way to transcend the onslaught of advice and experts, and switch on your intuition...

You must be willing to make mistakes.

You are kind and capable, and mothers have been successfully raising babies for a long time, long before books or the internet were invented.

You don't need to be rescued by an expert. You are the hero of your own motherhood adventure and you can find your own way out of the confusion by getting comfortable with the messy reality of motherhood, and getting hands-on with your baby.

You need to learn how to read your baby, not a book.

Every time you experiment with something new (which sometimes turns out to be a mistake), you are like a scientist reading the response, adjusting your course, gathering data on your baby and your parenting style. It's like getting a degree at university, then going on to do your masters, then your doctorate, all on the unique topic of Your Child.

Eventually, over time, you will become confident and figure out what works, for yourself and your baby. And you'll realise you don't need that manual after all.

4. Embrace Baby Brain

Yep, you've changed from the inside out. You are not just you plus baby; you are a whole new person too.

During pregnancy, when another soul quite literally invades your body, you are forced into a new way of knowing and understanding your self as distinct from other. You are one, in a very real way.

And often this pervades your whole life experience, not only your relationship with your baby. It changes the way you make decisions related to giving and receiving, and to protecting yourself. It changes your sense of who you are and how you behave, and your purpose in life.

Allow yourself some time to settle in to this unchartered territory.

Give yourself some space to find your feet in this new, feminine way of knowing and understanding the world. Boost your baby brain and enjoy the gooey, mushy haze. Relish your new emotional range and accept your sensitivity as a gift!

In spite of grey matter reductions and short-term memory loss (or even perhaps because of it!) your new brain is beautiful thing. Embrace it!

5. Ask for Help

Friendship is one thing, but you also need practical, physical help. Parenting is not a one-woman job. Traditionally, it was the work of your whole community, but it's unlikely this will happen without your initiative.

You'll have to gather your courage and ask for help.

126

Perhaps your first thought is that you have no one to ask, but often what this really means is you have no one you feel comfortable asking for help. Maybe you need to get more comfortable with asking.

If you are struggling, start with boosting your oxytocin — this will open you up to deeper connections.

And if you can't do it for yourself, do it for the movement. When you ask for help you pave the way for other mothers to receive more help too.

Consider this. When you ask for help, what is the worst that could happen?

Then if you don't ask for help, what is the worst that could happen?

Feel the fear, and ask for help anyway.

6. Love Conquers All

The golden rule of postpartum is Love Conquers All.

I know the real golden rule is 'do unto others as you would do unto yourself', but for many mothers, this needs to be reversed. We have no trouble being kind, generous and caring towards others. In fact, we expend all our energy making other people healthy and happy, even at the expense of our own health and happiness.

So right now, you may need to put some effort into doing for yourself as you would do for others!

Focus on love.

Love yourself as you love your baby.

If this doesn't come easily to you, start by listening to your body. It never lies. If you are exhausted and overwhelmed, it's time to start doing something different.

Don't blindly follow rules or routines if they aren't working for you. Forget about what you are allowed to do or what you should do. Don't worry too much about making small inevitable mistakes.

Peace and joy always take precedent.

It's likely your memory isn't working how it used to right now, so if you only remember one message from this book, make it this.

Do what brings you peace and joy.

About the Author

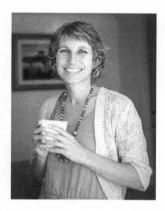

Julia Jones is a doula, author, entrepreneur and philanthropist.

She has trained hundreds of postpartum professionals around the world through her Australian College of Midwives recognised online course Newborn Mothers Collective.

She is the author of *Nourishing Newborn Mothers — Ayurvedic Recipes to Heal Your Mind, Body and Soul after Childbirth.*

She lives between the river and the ocean in her home town North Fremantle, with her husband, three children and pet rabbit.

Learn more at www.newbornmothers.com.

References

Introduction

1   Consultations.health.gov.au. (2018). Medicare Benefits
    Schedule Review Taskforce Consultation - Australian
    Government Department of Health - Citizen Space. [online]
    Available at: https://consultations.health.gov.au/medicare-
    reviews-unit/mbs-review/

2   Perrine, C. G., Scanlon, K. S., Li, R., Odom, E., & Grummer-
    Strawn, L. M. (2012). Baby- Friendly Hospital Practices and
    Meeting Exclusive Breastfeeding Intention. *PEDIATRICS,*
    130(1), 54–60. Retrieved from https://doi.org/10.1542/
    peds.2011-3633

3   Shapiro, A. F., & Gottman, J. M. (2005). Effects on Marriage
    of a Psycho- Communicative-Educational Intervention
    With Couples Undergoing the Transition to Parenthood,
    Evaluation at 1-Year Post Intervention. *Journal of Family*
    Communication, 5(1), 1–24. Retrieved from https://doi.
    org/10.1207/s15327698jfc0501_1

4   Lafrance, A. (2015). *What happens to a woman's brain*
    when she becomes a mother. Retrieved from https://www.
    theatlantic.com/health/archive/2015/01/what-happens-to-a-
    womans-brain-when-she-becomes-a-mother/384179/

Your Brain

1   Diamond, M. C., Johnson, R. E., & Ingham, C. (2009).
    Brain Plasticity Induced by Environment and Pregnancy,
    International *Journal of Neuroscience, 2*(4-5), 171-178.
    Retrieved from https://doi.org/10.3109/00207457109146999

2   Hoekzema, E., Barba-Müller, E., Pozzobon, C., Picado, M., Lucco, F., García-García, D., Soliva, J. C., Tobeña, A., Desco, M., Crone E. A., Ballesteros, A., Carmona, S., & Vilarroya, O. (2017). Pregnancy leads to long-lasting changes in human brain structure, *Nature Neuroscience, 20*(2), 287-300. Retrieved from https://doi.org/10.1038/nn.4458

3   Hillerer, K. M., Jacobs, V. R., Fischer, T., & Aigner, L. (2014). The maternal brain: An organ with peripartal plasticity. *Neural Plasticity*. Hindawi Publishing Corporation. https:// doi. org/10.1155/2014/574159

4   Klein, S. L, Schiebinger, L., Stefanick, M. L., Cahill, L. Danska, J., de Vries, G., Kibbe, M., McCarthy, M., Mogil, J., Woodruff, T., & Zucker, I. (2015). Opinion: Sex inclusion in basic research drives discovery: Fig. 1. *Proceedings of the Natural Academy of Sciences, 112*(17), 5257–5258. https:// doi.org/10.1073/pnas.1502843112

Learning

1   Wan, X., Nakatani, H., Ueno, K., Asamizuya, T., Cheng, K., & Tanaka, K. (2011). The neural basis of intuitive best next-move generation in board game experts, *Science, 331*(6015), 341-346. Retrieved from https://doi.org/10.1126/science.1194732

2   Hoekzema, E., Barba-Müller, E., Pozzobon, C., Picado, M., Lucco, F., García-García, D., Soliva, J. C., Tobeña, A., Desco, M., Crone E. A., Ballesteros, A., Carmona, S., & Vilarroya, O. (2017). Pregnancy leads to long-lasting changes in human brain structure, *Nature Neuroscience, 20*(2), 287-300. Retrieved from https://doi.org/10.1038/nn.4458

3   Hillerer, K. M., Jacobs, V. R., Fischer, T., & Aigner, L. (2014). The maternal brain: An organ with peripartal plasticity. *Neural Plasticity*. Hindawi Publishing Corporation. https:// doi. org/10.1155/2014/574159

Loving

1 Uvnäs Moberg, K. (2003). *The Oxytocin Factor: Tapping the Hormone of Calm, Love, and Healing*, Brixton: Pinter & Martin Publishers

2 Uvnäs Moberg, K. (2016). *Oxytocin: The Biological Guide to Motherhood*, Praeclarus Press

3 Petersson, M., Alster, P., Lundeberg, T., & Uvnäs-Moberg, K. (1996). Oxytocin increases nociceptive thresholds in a long-term perspective in female and male rats. *Neuroscience Letters, 212*(2), 87-90. Retrieved from https://doi. org/10.1016/0304-3940(96)12773-7

4 Uvnas-Moberg, K., & Petersson, M. (2005). Oxytocin, a mediator of anti-stress, well- being, social interaction, growth and healing. *Zeitschrift Für Psychosomatische Medizin Und Psychotherapie, 51*(1) [online]. Available at: https://doi.org/10 .3109/10253890.2011.631154

5 Argiolas, A., & Gessa, G. L. (1991). Central functions of oxytocin. *Neuroscience and Biobehavioral Reviews, 15*(2), 217-231. Retrieved from https://doi.org/10.1016/ S0149-7634(05)80002-8

6 Uvnäs-Moberg, K. (1998). Oxytocin may mediate the benefits of positive social interaction and emotions, *Psychoneuroendocrinology, 23*(8), 819–835. Retrieved from https://doi.org/10.1016/S0306-4530(98)00056-0

7 Uvnäs-Moberg, K. (1997). Physiological and endocrine effects of social contact, *Annals of the New York Academy of Sciences, 807,* 146–163. Retrieved from https://doi. org/10.1111/j.1749-6632.1997.tb51917.x

8 Uvnäs-Moberg, K. (1998). Antistress Pattern Induced by Oxytocin. *News in Physiological Sciences, 13*(2), 22–26. Retrieved from https://doi.org/10.1016/0304-3940(95)11335-t

9   Svennersten, K., Nelson, L., & Uvnäs-Moberg, K. (1990)
     Feeding-induced oxytocin release in dairy cows, *Acta
     Physiological Scandinavica, 140*(2), 295-296. Retrieved from
     https://doi.org/10.1111/j.1748-1716.1990.tb09001.x

10   Ekström, A., Widström, A., & Nissen, E. (2003).
     Breastfeeding Support from Partners and Grandmothers:
     Perceptions of Swedish Women, *Birth, 30*(4), 261-
     266. Retrieved from https://doi.org/10.1046/j.1523-
     536X.2003.00256.x

11   Emmott, E. H., & Mace, R. (2015). Practical support from
     fathers and grandmothers is associated with lower levels
     of breastfeeding in the UK millennium cohort study. *PLoS
     ONE, 10*(7). Retrieved from https://doi.org/10.1371/journal.
     pone.0133547

12   Grassley, J.S., Spencer, B.S., & Law, B. (2012). A
     grandmothers' tea: evaluation of a breastfeeding support
     intervention. *The Journal of Perinatal Education, 21*(2), 80-
     89. Retrieved from https://doi.org/10.1891/1058-1243.21.2.80

13   Braga, R. I., Panaitescu, A., Bădescu, S., Zăgrean, A. M., &
     Zăgrean, L. (2014). Intranasal administration of oxytocin
     alters sleep architecture. *Biological Rhythm Research, 45*(1),
     69–75. Retrieved from https://doi.org/10.1080/09291016.201
     3.797641

14   Shahrestani, S., Kemp, A. H., & Guastella, A. J. (2013). The
     impact of a single administration of intranasal oxytocin on the
     recognition of basic emotions in humans: A meta-analysis.
     Neuropsychopharmacology, 38(10), 1929–1936. Retrieved
     from https:// doi.org/10.1038/npp.2013.86

15 Olff, M., Frijling, J. L., Kubzansky, L. D., Bradley, B.,
     Ellenbogen, M. A., Cardoso, C., Bartz, J. A., Yee, J. R.,
     & van Zuiden, M. (2013). The role of oxytocin in social
     bonding, stress regulation and mental health: An update on the
     moderating effects of context and interindividual differences.

Psychoneuroendocrinology, 38(9), 1883–1894. Retrieved from https://doi.org/10.1016/j.psyneuen.2013.06.019

16 Kerstin Uvnäs Moberg. Retrieved from http://www.kerstinuvnasmoberg.com/kerstin- uvnas-moberg/

17 Zak, P J. (2001). *The Moral Molecule: The New Science of What Makes Us Good or Evil*, Penguin Publishing Group

Variety

1 Zak, P J. (2001). *The Moral Molecule: The New Science of What Makes Us Good or Evil*, Penguin Publishing Group

The Future

1 Ellison, K. (2005). *The Mommy Brain: How Motherhood Makes Us Smarter,* New York, NY: Basic Books

Your Village

1 Dunsworth, H. M. (2016). Thank your intelligent mother for your big brain. *Proceedings of the National Academy of Sciences, 113*(25), 816-6818. Retrieved from https://doi.org/10.1073/pnas.1606596113

2 Dunsworth, H. M. (2016). *Labor Pains and Helpless Infants: Eve or Evolution? (Part 1)*. Retrieved from https://www.sapiens.org/column/origins/labor-pains-helpless-infants-eve-evolution-part-one/

3 Dunsworth, H. M., Warrener, A. G., Deacon, T., Ellison, P. T., & Pontzer, H. (2012). Metabolic hypothesis for human altriciality. *Proceedings of the National Academy of Sciences, 109*(38), 15212–15216. Retrieved from https://doi.org/10.1073/pnas.1205282109

History

1   Blaffer Hrdy, S. (2011). *Mothers and Others: The Evolutionary Origins of Mutual Understanding*, Belknap Press.

2   Harkness, S. (2015) The Strange Situation of Attachment Research: A Review of Three Books, *Reviews in Anthropology, 44*(3), 178-197. Retrieved from https://doi.org/ 10.1080/00938157.2015.1088337

Traditions

1   Perrine, C. G., Scanlon, K. S., Li, R., Odom, E., & Grummer-Strawn, L. M. (2012). Baby- Friendly Hospital Practices and Meeting Exclusive Breastfeeding Intention. *PEDIATRICS, 130*(1), 54–60. Retrieved from https://doi.org/10.1542/peds.2011-3633

2   Raphael, D. (2007). *Breastfeeding and Doula Support.* Retrieved from https:// www.childresearch.net/aboutCS/researchers/2007_01.html

3   *Hygge.* (n.d) in English Oxford Living Dictionaries. Retrieved from https:// en.oxforddictionaries.com/definition/hygge

4   Ewaschuk, J. (2010). *The Scent of a Woman*, Mothering Publishing Inc

5   Dunman, C. & Aria, B. (1991). *Mamatoto: A Celebration of Birth*, Viking

6   Hoekzema, E., Barba-Müller, E., Pozzobon, C., Picado, M., Lucco, F., García-García, D., Solvia, J. C., Tobeña, A., Desco, M., Crone, E. A., Ballesteros, A., Carmona. S., & Vilarroya, O. (2017). Pregnancy leads to long-lasting changes in human brain structure. *Nature Neuroscience, 20*(2), 287–296. Retrieved from https://doi.org/10.1038/nn.4458

7   Woolhouse, H., Gartland, D., Mensah, F., & Brown, S. J.
    (2015). Maternal depression from early pregnancy to 4
    years postpartum in a prospective pregnancy cohort study:
    Implications for primary health care. *BJOG: An International
    Journal of Obstetrics and Gynaecology, 122*(3), 312–321.
    Retrieved from https://doi.org/10.1111/1471-0528.12837

8   Who. (2009). Mental health aspects of women's reproductive
    health. *World Health, 61*(4), 1–67. Retrieved from https://doi.
    org/10.1176/appi.ps.61.4.421